The Climate and COVID-19

The Climate and COVID-19:

Global Challenges and Responses

Edited by

Sultan Ayoub Meo
and Khalid Mahmood Shafi

Cambridge
Scholars
Publishing

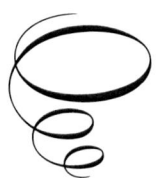

The Climate and COVID-19: Global Challenges and Responses

Edited by Sultan Ayoub Meo and Khalid Mahmood Shafi

This book first published 2022

Cambridge Scholars Publishing

Lady Stephenson Library, Newcastle upon Tyne, NE6 2PA, UK

British Library Cataloguing in Publication Data
A catalogue record for this book is available from the British Library

ISBN (10): 1-5275-8606-5
ISBN (13): 978-1-5275-8606-2

Contents

Preface

During the past two decades, there has been a significant shift in social demographics; people are shifting from rural to urban regions resulting in a swift upward shift in the urban population. This rapid, unplanned urbanization and industrialization has contributed to environmental pollution. Urbanization and industrialization are major contributing factors to the ongoing change in the global climate. The environment and weather conditions have a great effect on the pattern of human health and diseases.

The "Severe Acute Respiratory Syndrome Coronavirus 2 (SARS-CoV-2)," also known as the COVID-19 pandemic, has also been linked with weather conditions and environmental pollution. The present pandemic has caused a global public health crisis with long-lasting economic damage. The situation and the lockdown have affected people's social and psychological health, from all ages and walks of life. The young generations who have been exposed will remember it, and be adversely affected by it, for many years. COVID-19 and climate change have collectively demonstrated that the most commanding and influential force on earth is the established natural sciences of biology, chemistry and physics versus the artificial and lust-based human targets of business and economies. The climate crisis and COVID-19 pandemic are a portal for the world. We have the option to go through it with our deeds, and conventional and traditional notions. The health, stability, and strength of future generations depend on the collective concepts of sharing and caring for our beautiful planet.

This book highlights the journey from the fog of a pandemic into the storm of climate change, that is challenging humanity. The contributors to this volume have amply highlighted the assorted aspects of this highly challenging and threatening situation of climate and the COVID-19 pandemic. The authors have covered wide-ranging topics associated with medicine, environment, weather conditions, environmental pollution, human rights, and political and emerging global scenarios. The authors of this book aim to highlight the complex dimensions of the COVID-19 pandemic and emphasize the need to synchronize the social and political order.

The global community should be prepared for COVID and climate aspects for pre-emptive policies. Suppose a single virus can smear out the huge economy in a year and completely lock down societies. In that case, this is a testimony to the fact that economies and communities are not very buoyant.

Global leaders have to understand the magnitude of such pandemics, climate crises, and conventional conflicts of the assorted aspects of human security.

Authors and contributors

Acknowledgements

This book would not have been possible without the support of family, friends, and colleagues. First of all, we are thankful to our family members and children for their immense support which helped us to concentrate on the book manuscripts with dedication. We are grateful to our Institutes: College of Medicine, King Saud University, Riyadh, Saudi Arabia; National Defence University, Islamabad, Pakistan; Mills-Peninsula Medical Center, South San Mateo, California, USA; University of Health Sciences, Lahore, Pakistan; National University of Medical Sciences (NUMS), Rawalpindi, Pakistan, and School of Law, Cardiff University, Cardiff, UK.

We owe our special thanks to Prof. Muhamad Mujahid Khan, Professor of Cell Biology and Anatomy, Dar Al Uloom University, Riyadh, KSA, and Mr. Rana Ather Javaid, Mr. Arif, and Mr. Tahir, Mr. Adnan Mehmood Usmani, for their support.

We are also thankful to Ms. Helen Edwards, and Cambridge Scholars Publishing, for their support while publishing our book.

Editors, Authors, and contributors

Contributors

1. **Prof. Sultan Ayoub Meo**

   MBBS, Ph.D. (Pak), M Med Ed (Dundee), FRCP (London), FRCP (Dublin), FRCP (Glasgow), FRCP (Edinburgh).
   Professor and Consultant in Clinical Physiology, Department of Physiology, King Khalid University Hospital, College of Medicine, King Saud University, Riyadh, Saudi Arabia.

2. **Dr Khalid Mahmood Shafi**

   Ph.D., M Phil, MSc, MA (Hons)
   National Defence University, Islamabad, Pakistan

3. **Prof. David C. Klonoff**

   M.D., FACP, FRCP (Edin), Fellow AIMBE
   President, Diabetes Technology Society, USA
   Clinical Professor of Medicine, U.C. San Francisco
   Editor-in-Chief, Journal of Diabetes Science and Technology
   Medical Director, Diabetes Research Institute
   Mills-Peninsula Medical Center, 100 South San Mateo Drive, Room 5147
   San Mateo, California 94401

4. **Prof. Javed Akram**

   MRCP (U.K.), FRCP (London), FRCP (Glasgow),
   FRCP (Edin), FACC (USA), FACP (USA), FASIM (USA)
   Professor of Medicine and Vice-Chancellor
   University of Health Sciences, Khayaban-e-Jamia, Lahore, Punjab, 54600, Pakistan

5. **Prof. Nadia Naseem, MBBS, M.Phil, Ph.D.**

   Professor, Department of Morbid Anatomy and Histopathology,
   University of Health Sciences, Khayaban-e-Jamia, Lahore, Punjab, 54600
   Pakistan

6. **Dr. Anusha Sultan Meo, MBBS**

   Army Medical College, National University of Medical Sciences (NUMS) Rawalpindi, Pakistan

7. **Barrister Tehreem Sultan, LLB (UK), BPTC (Lincoln's Inn, London, UK)**

   Trainee, International Criminal Court, Hague, Netherlands

8. **Ruhaab Khalid, LLB**

   School of Law, Cardiff University, Cardiff, UK

Brief Biography

Prof. Sultan Ayoub Meo

MBBS, Ph.D. (Pak), M Med Ed (Dundee), FRCP (London), FRCP (Dublin), FRCP (Glasgow), FRCP (Edinburgh).

Professor Meo is a professor and consultant in Clinical Physiology, Department of Physiology, King Khalid University Hospital, College of Medicine, King Saud University, Riyadh, Saudi Arabia. Prof Meo is credited with ten books and over 190 scientific papers in peer-reviewed national/ International, pub-med, and Web of Science indexed bio-medical Journals.

Professor Meo has been appointed as a Ph.D. supervisor and examiner in various universities of Saudi Arabia and Malaysia. In an Editorial capacity, Prof Meo served as an Associate Editor of many Web of Science Indexed international journals. Prof Meo has been invited as a speaker and keynote speaker to deliver the talk in more than 125 National / International conferences in different states, including Pakistan, Saudi Arabia, Bahrain, United Arab Emirates, China, Turkey, Indonesia, United Kingdom, and the USA. Prof. Meo received an Excellency award in Medicine in the year 2017.

Dr. Khalid Mahmood Shafi

Ph.D, M Phil, MSc, MA (Hons)

Dr. Khalid is an academician and a practitioner with over thirty years of field experience. His main areas of specialization include Climate Change, Global policy, and Security Sector reforms. He has served in a field where in addition to an active leadership role in peacebuilding operations, he has contributed to disaster risk management and people-centric sustainable development. He has written articles in national and international journals on topics of Policy reforms, Climate Change, Air Pollution, COVID-19, Civil Society, UN, Peacebuilding, and environmental issues in the Global South. He has also served in United Nations. His second book titled, "UN, Pakistan and Climate crisis" is under publication..

Prof. David C. Klonoff

M.D., FACP, FRCP (Edin), Fellow AIMBE

Prof. David C Klonoff is an endocrinologist specializing in diabetes technology. He is the Medical Director of the Dorothy L. and James E. Frank Diabetes Research Institute of Mills-Peninsula Health Services in San Mateo, California, and a Clinical Professor of Medicine at UCSF. Dr. Klonoff graduated from UC Berkeley; his postgraduate training included two years at UCLA Hospital and three years at UCSF Hospitals. Dr. Klonoff is cited as among the top 1% of U.S. endocrinologists by Castle Connolly Medical Ltd. He received an FDA Director's Special Citation Award in 2010 for outstanding contributions to diabetes technology. In 2012 Dr. Klonoff was elected a Fellow of the American Institute of Medical and Biological Engineering and cited as among the top 2% of bioengineers worldwide. He received the 2012 Gold Medal Oration and Distinguished Scientist Award from the Mohan's Diabetes Specialties Centre and Madras Diabetes Research Foundation of Chennai, India. He was elected a Fellow of the Royal College of Physicians (Edinburgh) in 2015. Dr. Klonoff has advised FDA and FTC, grant review for NIH, CDC, NASA, NSF, U.S. Army, ADA, JDRF, and five foreign governments. He has been invited to scientific meetings at the White House and the European Parliament. He is the author of dozens of books, book chapters, and over 250 research articles.

Prof. Javed Akram

MRCP(U.K.), FRCP(London), FRCP(Glasgow),

FRCP(Edin), FACC(USA), FACP(USA), FASIM(USA)

Prof Javed Akram is an eminent Professor of Medicine, outstanding physician, renowned medical educationist, innovative researcher, and policymaker in Pakistan. He is an author of six medical books and over 100 research papers and supervised over 120 postgraduate students. Prof. Akram graduated from King Edward Medical College, Lahore, in 1979. He completed his postgraduate training from RCP (U.K.). He obtained a Fellowship of the Royal College of Physicians of London, Glasgow, and Edinburgh. He served as the Principal of Allama Iqbal Medical College and the Chief Executive Jinnah Hospital, Lahore. He was elevated as Vice-Chancellor (Rector) of Shaheed Zulfiqar Ali Bhutto Medical University, Islamabad, and CEO of the Pakistan Institute of Medical Sciences (PIMS). After that, he was appointed as Vice-Chancellor, University of Health Sciences (UHS) Lahore, where he is currently working. In recognition of his clinical and community services, the president of Pakistan awarded him with a civil award, "Tamgha-e-Imtiaz."

Prof. Nadia Naseem

MBBS, M.Phil, Ph.D.

Professor, Department of Morbid Anatomy and Histopathology, University of Health Sciences (UHS), Lahore, Pakistan
She has teaching experience of about two decades in medical universities. She is an Editor In-chief of Bio-Medica journal, University of Health Sciences (UHS), Lahore. She is credited with over 100 research articles in peer-reviewed national and international biomedical journals.

Dr. Anusha Sultan Meo, MBBS

Army Medical College, National University of Medical Sciences (NUMS), Rawalpindi, Pakistan.
Anusha is a research-oriented young physician, currently completing her internship. She has authored dozens of research articles in different web of science indexed science journals. During her university tenure, she won multiple awards at different debating/writing competitions and MUNs, later which she also chaired and presided over. She has also served as the President of the Debates and Literary Society at Army Medical College.

Barrister Tehreem Sultan, LLB (UK), BPTC (Lincoln's Inn, London, UK), Trainee, International Criminal Court, Hague, Netherlands

Barrister Tehreem Sultan is a First Class Law Graduate with a particular interest in Criminal and International Human Rights Law. She is currently working as an intern at the International Criminal Court. She has been actively involved in the criminal justice system and is the Director for the UK award winning prison teaching programme, Vocalise. She frequently writes for the Oxford Human Rights Hub, UK Human Rights Blog.

Ruhaab Khalid, LLB

School of Law, Cardiff University, Cardiff, UK

Ms. Ruhaab is a young, motivated writer and law student at Cardiff University, U.K. She has written articles in journals such as Cardiff Law Review and Pakistan Horizon. She has been working on climate change-associated research articles in one of the leading newspapers of Wales, the Gairrhydd. Currently, she is a research advocate at the organizations of Hope and Victim Support.

COVID-19 Pandemic: Biological and Epidemiological Trends

Sultan Ayoub Meo

Abstract

The Severe Acute Respiratory Syndrome Coronavirus-2 (SARS-CoV-2) infection outbreak has posed a significant threat to the global health care system and economy. The novel coronavirus, also known as the COVID-19 pandemic, is highly contagious and has affected over 110 million people worldwide, with a mortality of about 2.4 million. The disease is swiftly spreading, with fluctuating prevalence and mortality trends. Regional and international health officials have taken priority measures to prevent further outbreaks of this emerging pathogen across the globe and to minimize the prevalence and mortality. However, the growing number of cases and deaths is demonstrating a need to further enhance public health mediations, vaccinations, good hygiene conditions, social distancing, use of masks, and movement limitations in order to control the COVID-19 pandemic. This manuscript highlights the biological and epidemiological trends of SARS-CoV-2.

Keywords: Coronavirus, SARS-CoV-2, COVID-19 pandemic, Epidemiology

Introduction

Over the past two decades, worldwide, people have been facing several infectious disease outbreaks, including Ebola, Influenza A (H1N1), Severe Acute Respiratory Syndrome Coronavirus (SARS), Middle East Respiratory Syndrome (MERS), and the Zika virus. Most recently, the global outbreak of novel coronavirus 2019, also known as Severe Acute Respiratory Syndrome Coronavirus-2 (SARS-CoV-2), has enhanced to a globally threatening pandemic [1]. SARS-CoV-2, also known as the COVID-19 pandemic, is a highly contagious infection, reported for the first time in Wuhan, China, in Dec 2019 [2]. The SARS-CoV-2 infection has spread through transmission from animal to animal, animal to human, and human-to-human, through droplets, via direct or indirect contact, culminating in a devastating pandemic [3].

The recent outbreak of the COVID-19 pandemic has caused a severe global threat. As per the World Health Organization (WHO) report on February

18, 2021, the novel coronavirus has affected over 110 million people, with a mortality of about 2.4 million people worldwide. In March 2020, the World Health Organization declared the COVID-19 outbreak a pandemic [4]. The disease is diffusing across the world has crossed all the earlier statistical facts and figures. [5]. The global evidence indicates its initial circulation in bats, before transmitting via an intermediate host to humans [3]. The risk of a reverse spread from companion animals to humans could also increase the risk of COVID-19 infection and its chances of mutation [6]. The science community is facing the challenging issue of further mutations, and the prevalence and mortality have not settled down.

Biology of the Novel Coronavirus

Coronaviruses belong to the family "Coronaviridae" and "subfamily Coronavirinae". Coronaviruses are classified into four genera: "Alpha, Beta, Gamma, and Delta coronavirus" [7]. SARS-CoV-2 is a highly pathogenic coronavirus that emerged among human populations. The previous coronaviruses that have affected humans are: "the Middle East Respiratory Syndrome Coronavirus (MERS-CoV), coronaviruses (HCoVs) including HCoV-229E, HCoV-NL63, HCoV-OC43, and HCoV-HKU1". These viruses have been scattered in the human population for hundreds of years and cause mild respiratory illness, with 5-30% having clinical features like the common cold [8].

Table 1.1: Biological Characteristics of Coronavirus.

Family: Coronaviridae
Subfamily: Coronavirinae
Types: Alpha, Beta, Gamma, and Delta coronavirus
Coronavirus: Round, globular, oval, elliptic in shape with a size of about 60 to 220 nm
Toroviruses: Kidney or rod-shaped, disk-like in appearance with a size of about 120 to 140 nm
Envelope: Envelope in large, widely spaced club-shaped peplomers
RNA Genome: Linear, plus sense ssRNA genome 27 to 33 kb, polyadenylated sequences
Structural proteins: "Nucleoprotein (N)," "Peplomer glycoprotein (S)," "Transmembrane glycoprotein (M)," and "Hemagglutinin-esterase (HE)."
The genome encodes three to ten non-structural proteins.
Replication: Replicates in the cytoplasm [9, 10]

The coronaviruses are positive-strand RNA viruses, with an approximate size of about 60-220 nm. The biological features are a crown-like appearance due to spike glycoproteins radiating from the virus envelope [9, 10]. Coronaviruses virions contain three major structural proteins. The very large 200 K glycoprotein S for a spike provides large 15-20 nm peplomers in the viral envelope. The second one is a transmembrane glycoprotein (M), and the third one is an internal phosphorylated nucleocapsid protein (N). There is also a minor transmembrane protein E, and some coronaviruses contain envelope protein with hemagglutination and esterase functions [9, 11].

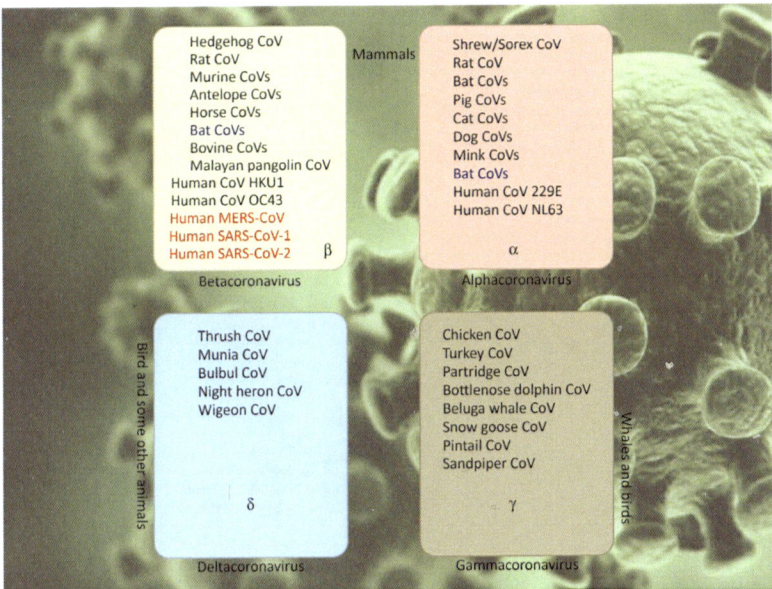

Figure 1.1: Phylogeny of coronaviruses.

Transmission Trends of Coronavirus

Coronaviruses may be found in a highly diverse range of different mammalian and bird host species. The combined impact of swift and unplanned urbanization, industrialization, farming, transportation systems, and climate change have provided a multiplicity of routes for coronaviruses to spill over into human populations [11-13]. In particular, a large proportion of coronaviruses are thought to reside in bats and seafood reservoirs, which are particularly adept at facilitating cross-species transmission [11]. Coronaviruses can easily circulate through various avian and mammalian species and reservoirs, including "bats, birds, cats, dogs, pigs, rodents, and humans" [14]. The global population has a long history of contagious infectious diseases by a coronavirus. The viral infections are highly contagious and easily spread through inhalation or ingestion of viral droplets during close communication or gathering, coughing, sneezing, and direct or indirect touching of infected surfaces with primary sources of infection [1].

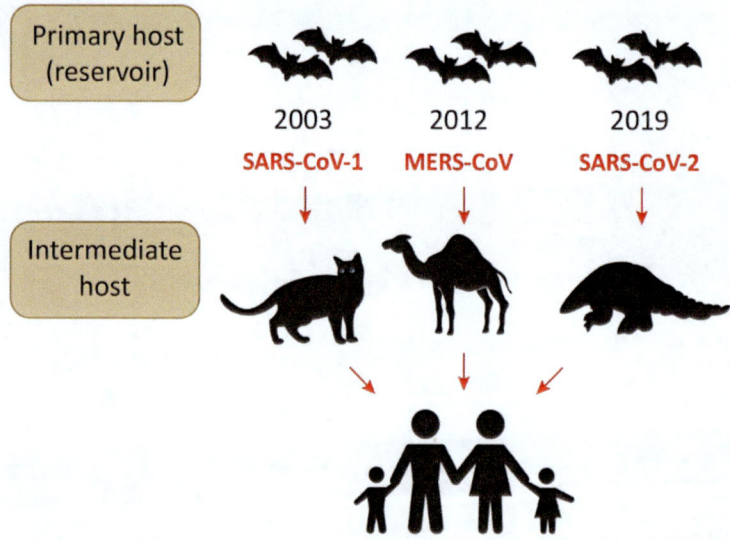

Figure 1.2: Transmission of coronavirus SARS-CoV-1, MERS-CoV, and SARS-CoV-2 infection.

The human respiratory system is highly vulnerable to infectious diseases. Pulmonary infections are transmitted through respiratory droplets. The droplet particles, with a size of about 5-10 μm or more in diameter, are known as respiratory droplets. On the other hand, droplets smaller than five μm in diameter are called "droplet nuclei" [15]. SARS-CoV-2 is mainly transmitted in people through respiratory droplets and direct and indirect contact routes. The transmission of droplets occurs when people are in close contact of about 1 meter with people who are suffering from SARS-CoV-2 infection, with or without respiratory symptoms. The chances of exposure to respiratory droplets are high during a close gathering, communication, coughing, or sneezing. These droplets can stay in the environment and, therefore, can easily spread from person to person [16].

The transmission of SARS-CoV-2 can occur through direct contact with infected people, or indirect contact with surfaces in the immediate environment [17], or with the kinds of stuff used by the infected person [15]. There is some evidence that SARS-CoV-2 infection involves the gastrointestinal system, causing intestinal disease, and the virus presents in feces, and may spread through fecal-oral and aerosol-borne routes [18].

The air pollutants, mainly particulate matter (PM) with a size of about PM2.5, enter into the human body, and are absorbed by human tissues or dissolved in body fluids based on their hydrophilic and hydrophobic characteristics. Environmental pollutants, particulate matter (PM2.5), constitute a significant risk factor for exaggerating the transmission of SARS-CoV-2 and markedly impairing human health [19]. More recently, it has also been reported that people prone, and exposed, to a high concentration of environmental pollution, PM2.5, are at increased risk of developing chronic respiratory diseases, including SARS-CoV-2 infection and mortality [20, 21]. Exposure to environmental pollutants, PM 2.5, carbon monoxide (CO), and ozone (O_3) increases the susceptibility to infections that damage human airways and potentially facilitate viral infections. Exposure to environmental pollution, PM2.5 pollutants, impairs the human immune system by decreasing the human body's ability to fight against viral infections, including the SARS-CoV-2 infection. The literature shows that outdoor and indoor pollutants, including PM2.5, carbon monoxide (CO), nitrogen dioxide (NO_2), and ozone (O_3), contribute to more severe SARS-CoV-2 infection and mortality. These facts demonstrate that various biological and physical factors spread the SARS-CoV-2 infection [20].

Epidemiological Trends of SARS-CoV-2 Infection

Since the appearance of the first case of SARS-CoV-2 infection in Wuhan, China, the spread of the disease has not settled down. The biological and epidemiological trends in the prevalence and mortality rate are swiftly changing on a daily basis. Initially, China was the disease's epicenter, but the disease was transmitted worldwide within 6-8 weeks. The disease burden was gradually transmitted and increased in other states, mainly Europe and the United States of America. Despite all the recent collective efforts, the COVID-19 pandemic is a highly challenging virus for the science community, policymakers, and the general public.

Meo et al., 2020 [22] conducted a study on the rising trends in the transmission, prevalence, and mortality rate due to COVID-19. The current epidemiological trends demonstrate that COVID-19 is highly contagious and has involved 109,594,835 people globally, with a mortality rate of 2,244,060 (2.21%) [4]. The authors reported the epidemiological trends from December 29, 2019, to March 31, 2020. During the study period, worldwide, the total number of infected cases was 750,890, resulting in 36,405 deaths with a mortality rate of 4.84%. The infection was more common in males over 60 years of age. The mean growth factor for the total number of cases from January 23 to March 31, 2020, was 1.20, and the growth factor for mortality was 1.12 [22].

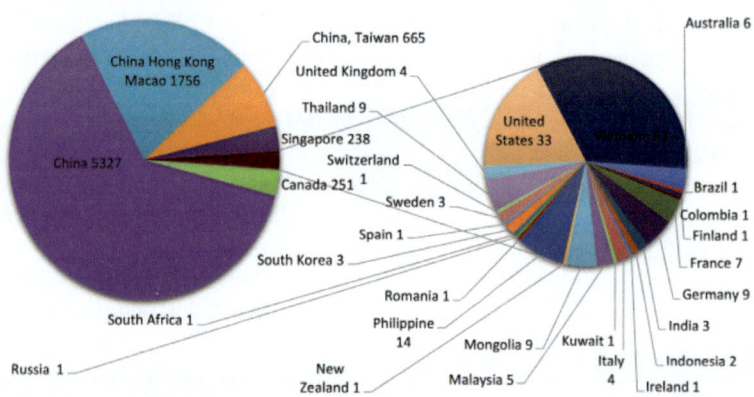

Figure 1.3: SARS-CoV-1 data presented from November 2002 to August 2003 [Figure adopted after permission from author and publisher] [2].

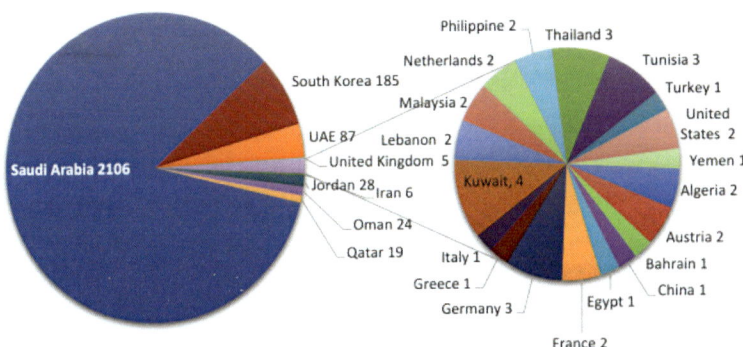

Figure 1.4: Worldwide prevalence of Middle East Respiratory Syndrome Coronavirus (MERS-CoV) infection.
Note: MERS-CoV data presented from June 2012 to February 7, 2020 [Figure adopted after permission from author and publisher] [2].

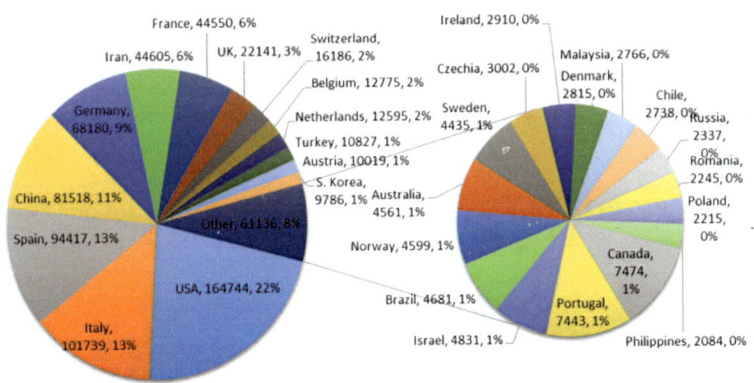

Figure 1.5: Worldwide prevalence of SARS-CoV-2.
The data was presented from December 29, 2019, to March 31, 2020. [Adopted after permission from author and publisher] [22].

After one year of this study, the number of SARS-CoV-2 confirmed cases are 109,594,835 with a mortality rate of 2,244,060 (2.21%) [4]. The findings suggest that the number of SARS-CoV-2 cases is continuously rising; however, the mortality rate decreases [Figures 1.6 and 1.7].

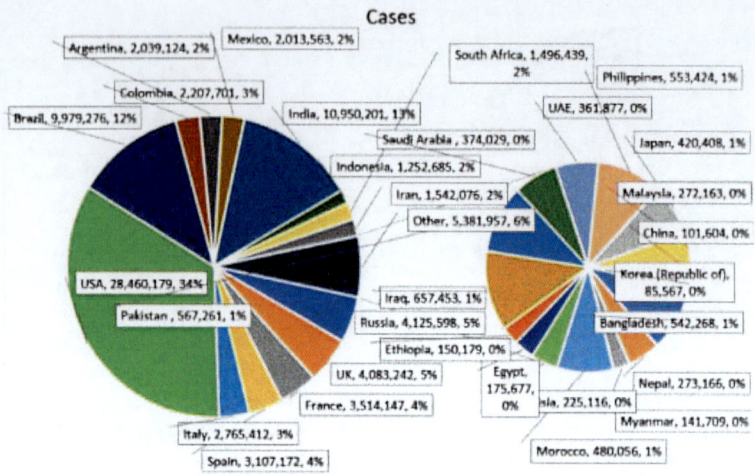

Figure 1.6: The worldwide cases of COVID-19 pandemic [Figure based on WHO data, February 18, 2021] [4].

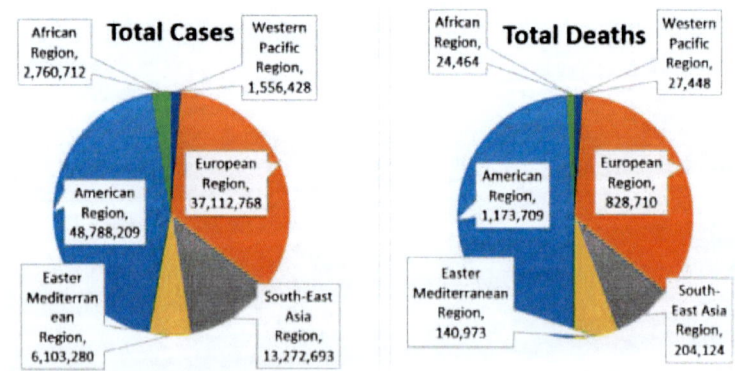

Figure 1.7: Worldwide cases and deaths due to COVID-19 pandemic [Figure based on WHO data, February 18, 2021] [4].

Table 1.2: Biological characteristics of coronavirus: 2019-nCoV, MERS-CoV and SARS-CoV

Characteristics	2019-nCoV	SARS-CoV	MERS-CoV
	Biological Characteristics		
Incubation period	2-14 (5.2) days	2-10 (7) days	2-10 (5.5) days
The median age of affected individuals	59 years	65 years	50 years
Male / Female	Male predominance	Male predominance	Male predominance
Virus	Positive-sense single-stranded RNA	Positive-sense single-stranded RNA	Positive-sense single-stranded RNA
Source of Origin	Seafood, snake, bats	Bats, civet cats	Bats, camel
Transmission	Animal-human human-human Zoonotic disease	Animal-Human Human-Human Zoonotic disease	Animal-human/ Human-Human Zoonotic disease
Speed of spread	High	Moderate	Low
Seasonal occurrence	Winter (Dec-Jan)	Winter (Dec-Jan)	Summer (May-July)
	Clinical Characteristics		
Headache	+	+	+
Fever	++	++	++
Chills or rigors	++	++	++
Generalized myalgia	++	++	++
Malaise	+	+	+
Drowsy	+	+	+
Confusion	+	+	+
	Pulmonary characteristics		
Dyspnea	+	+	+
Cough	++	++	++

Shortness of breath	+	+	+
Pneumonia	++	++	++
Hemoptysis	+	+	+
	Extra-pulmonary characteristics		
Abdominal pain	+/-	+/-	+/-
Nausea and vomiting	+	+	+
Diarrhea	+/-	+/-	+/-
Acute renal failure	+/-	+/-	+/-
	Blood analysis		
White Blood Cells count			
Lymphocytes count			
Platelets count			
Red Blood Cells count			
Overall fatality	2.11%	10.77%	34.77%

[+Mild; ++ Moderate; +++ severe; ⇧increase; ⇩decrease; +/- on and off]
[Table adopted after permission from author and publisher] [2].

The patterns of SARS-CoV-2, SARS-CoV-1, and MERS-CoV infections have been observed to have seasonal variations. Nassar and Meo et al., 2020 [2] reported that the outbreak of MERS-CoV was mainly during the summer period. The highest global seasonal occurrence of the MERS-CoV outbreak was found in June, while the lowest prevalence of disease was found in January from 2012 to 2017 [2]. In comparison, the SARS-CoV-1 and SARS-CoV-2 infection outbreaks took place mainly in winter weather (Table 1.2). The outbreak of this novel coronavirus "2019-nCoV" has been seen in the winter season, in strong contrast to the outbreaks of MERS-CoV. The gender-based analysis demonstrates that the cases mainly consisted of men with a median age range of 50-65 years [4, 13]. The virus mainly occurred among older people with a median age of 59 years.

There is heterogeneity in the transmissibility of "2019-nCoV, SARS, and MERS" outbreaks and, in particular, the occurrence of super-spreading events. The 2019-nCoV spread faster than the events of the previous epidemics "SARS-CoV-1, and MERS-CoV". SARS-CoV-1 spread into 32 countries, with 8,422 confirmed cases from November 2002 to August 2003. MERS-CoV spread over 27 states, resulting in 2,496 cases from April 2012 to February 7, 2020 [2]. However, the novel coronavirus SARS-CoV-2 spread worldwide and infected 109,594,835 people with a mortality rate of 2,424,060 (2.21%) from December 29, 2019, to February 17, 2021 [4]. The SARS-CoV-2 coronavirus is still in its spreading phase.

The clinical appearances of 2019-nCoV, SARS-CoV, and MERS-CoV infections cover a wide-ranging spectrum fluctuating from asymptomatic presentation and mild to severe acute respiratory illness, to death [2]. A distinctive presentation of these coronavirus symptoms is "fever of 38°C or more, fever with chills or rigors, generalized myalgia, malaise, drowsiness, confusion, dyspnea, coughing, shortness of breath and a radiological pulmonary presentation of pneumonia" (Table 1.2). The extra-pulmonary features include "abdominal disorders, nausea, vomiting, headache, diarrhea, neurological features, and acute renal failure." The other laboratory-based findings are an "increase in white blood cells, mainly neutrophils, and a decrease in lymphocytes, platelets, and red blood cells." The novel coronavirus, SARS-CoV-2, is highly contagious with various biological and epidemiological trends.

Conclusion

SARS-CoV-2 is highly contagious compared to earlier coronaviruses and has affected a large number of people worldwide. The infection has mainly affected older individuals and people with chronic debilitating diseases such as diabetes mellitus, cardiovascular diseases, and malignancy. International health officials have taken high-priority preventive measures to stop the outbreak of this emerging pathogen across the globe. However, SARS-CoV-2 is swiftly spreading, with mutable biological trends and rising epidemiological incidence. The rising epidemiological facts and figures are signifying a need to enhance the public health mediations, vaccination, good hygienic conditions, social distancing, and movement limitations, in order to control the COVID-19 epidemic across the globe.

References

1. Boopathi S, Poma AB, Kolandaivel P. Novel 2019 coronavirus structure, mechanism of action, antiviral drug promises and rule out against its treatment [published online ahead of print, 2020 April 30]. J Biomol Struct Dyn. 2020;1-10. doi:10.1080/07391102.2020.1758788

2. Meo S.A., Alhowaikan A., Al-khlaiwi T., Meo I.M., Halepoto D.M., Iqbal M., Usmani A.M., Hajjar W., Ahmed N. Novel coronavirus 2019-nCoV: prevalence, biological and clinical characteristics comparison with SARS-CoV and MERS-CoV. Eur. Rev. Med. Pharmacol. Sci. 2020;24(4):2012–2019.

3. Ng LFP, Hiscox JA. Coronaviruses in animals and humans. BMJ. 2020 Feb 19; 368():m634.

4. World Health Organization. Coronavirus Dashboard. Available at: https://covid19.who.int/. Cited date February 18, 2021.

5. Guo YR, Cao QD, Hong ZS, Tan YY, Chen SD, Jin HJ, Tan KS, Wang DY, Yan Y. The origin, transmission, and clinical therapies on coronavirus disease 2019 (COVID-19) outbreak an update on the status. Mil Med Res. 2020; 7 (1): 11.

6. Singla R, Mishra A, Joshi R, et al. Human-animal interface of SARS-CoV-2 (COVID-19) transmission: a critical appraisal of scientific evidence. Vet Res Commun. 2020;44(3-4):119-130. doi:10.1007/s11259-020-09781-0

7. De Groot R. Family – Coronaviridae. In: King AMQ, Adams MJ, Carstens EB, Lefkowitz EJ, editors. Virus Taxonomy. Elsevier; 2012. p. 806-828.

8. Corman VM, Muth D, Niemeyer D. Chapter eight - hosts and sources of endemic human coronaviruses. In: Kielian M, Mettenleiter TC, Roossinck MJ, editors. Advances in virus research. 100: Academic Press; 2018. p. 163-188.

9. Burrell CJ, Howard CR, Murphy FA. Coronaviruses. Fenner and White's Medical Virology. 2017;437-446. doi:10.1016/B978-0-12-375156-0.00031-X

10. Maheswari S, Pethannan R, Sabarimurugan S. Air pollution enhances susceptibility to novel coronavirus (COVID-19) infection - an impact study. Environ Anal Health Toxicol. 2020 Dec;35 (4):e2020020-0. doi: 10.5620/eaht.2020020.

11. Lin-FaWang, Danielle E Anderson. Viruses in bats and potential spillover to animals and humans. Current Opinion in Virology. 2019; 34; 79-89.

12. Allen T, Murray KA, Zambrana-Torrelio C, Morse SS, Rondinini C, Di Marco M, Breit N, Olival KJ, Daszak P. Global hotspots and correlates of emerging zoonotic diseases. Nat Commun, 2017; 8: 1124

13. Meo SA, Abukhalaf AA, Alomar AA, Aljudi TW, Bajri HM, Sami W, Akram J, Akram SJ, Hajjar W. Impact of weather conditions on incidence and mortality COVID-19 pandemic in Africa. Eur Rev Med Pharmacol Sci. 2020 Sep;24(18):9753-9759. doi: 10.26355/eurrev_202009_23069. PMID: 33015822.

14. Perlman S, Netland J. Coronaviruses post-SARS: update on replication and pathogenesis. Nat Rev Microbiol 2009;7: 439-450.

15. World Health Organization (WHO). Modes of transmission of the virus causing COVID-19: implications for IPC precaution recommendations; Available from https://www.who.int/news-room/commentaries/detail/modes-of-transmission-of-virus-causing-covid-19-implications-for-ipc-precaution-recommendations. Cited February 12, 2021.

16. Huang C, Wang Y, Li X. Clinical features of patients infected with 2019 novel coronavirus in Wuhan, China. Lancet 2020;395: 497-506.

17. Ong SW, Tan YK, Chia PY, Lee TH, Ng OT, Wong MS. Air, surface environmental, and personal protective equipment contamination by severe acute respiratory syndrome coronavirus 2 (SARS-CoV-2) from the asymptomatic patient. JAMA 2020; 323(16):1610-1612. doi: 10.1001/jama.2020.3227

18. Arslan M, Xu B, Gamal El-Din M. Transmission of SARS-CoV-2 via fecal-oral and aerosols-borne routes: Environmental dynamics and implications for wastewater management in underprivileged societies. Sci Total Environ. 2020; 743:140709. doi: 10.1016/j.scitotenv.2020.140709.

19. Falcon-Rodriguez CI, Osornio-Vargas AR, Sada-Ovalle I, Segura-Medina P. Aeroparticles, composition, and lung diseases. Front Immunol 2016;7: 3.

20. Meo SA, Abukhalaf AA, Alomar AA, Alessa OM, Sami W, Klonoff DC. Effect of environmental pollutants PM-2.5, carbon monoxide, and ozone on the incidence and mortality of SARS-COV-2 infection in ten wildfire-affected counties in California. Sci Total Environ. 2021 Feb 25;757:143948. doi: 10.1016/j.scitotenv.2020.143948.

21. Meo SA, Abukhalaf AA, Alomar AA, Alessa OM. Wildfire and COVID-19 pandemic: effect of environmental pollution PM-2.5 and carbon monoxide on the dynamics of daily cases and deaths due to SARS-COV-2 infection in San-Francisco USA. Eur Rev Med Pharmacol Sci. 2020 Oct;24(19):10286-10292. doi: 10.26355/eurrev_202010_23253.

22. Meo SA, Al-Khlaiwi T, Usmani AM, Meo AS, Klonoff DC, Hoang TD. Biological and epidemiological trends in the prevalence and mortality due to outbreaks of novel coronavirus COVID-19. J King Saud Univ Sci. 2020;32(4):2495-2499. doi:10.1016/j.jksus.2020.04.004

Climate and the COVID-19 Pandemic: Effects of Heat and Humidity

Chapter 02

Sultan Ayoub Meo | Javed Akram

Abstract

The "Severe Acute Respiratory Syndrome Coronavirus 2 (SARS-CoV-2)" infection, also known as the COVID-19 pandemic, has swiftly involved the entire world with devastating consequences. The COVID-19 pandemic has caused a global public health crisis with long-lasting social, psychological, and economic damage. The weather-related dynamics have an impact on the pattern of human health and disease. This chapter highlights the effects of climate, heat, and humidity on daily case incidences and the mortality rates due to the COVID-19 pandemic in various world regions. In countries with high temperatures and low humidity, the mean daily case incidences, cumulative cases, and cumulative deaths were low compared to low temperatures and high humidity. Moreover, COVID-19 cases and fatalities per million population were significantly lower in countries with high temperatures than countries with low temperatures. The findings on the weather changes and epidemiological trends of the COVID-19 pandemic have aftermaths for policymakers and health officials.

Keywords: COVID-19 Pandemic, Climate, Temperature, Heat, Humidity, Incidence, Mortality

Introduction

The Severe Acute Respiratory Syndrome Coronavirus 2 (SARS-CoV-2) infection, also more famously known as the COVID-19 pandemic, has caused global damage to human health, lives, and socio-economic conditions [1]. The COVID-19 pandemic has been highly predominant and more devastating than some previous pandemics, such as the "Severe Acute Respiratory Syndrome Coronavirus (SARS-CoV-1) and the Middle East Respiratory Syndrome Coronavirus (MERS-CoV)" [2]. On February 12, 2021, worldwide it involved 216 countries and infected 107,423,526 people with a mortality rate of 2,360,280 (1.19%) [3].

The biological and epidemiological trends in the prevalence and mortality rates due to the COVID-19 pandemic are swiftly changing. Initially, China bore the largest burden of the coronavirus, but the incidence is gradually increasing in other countries, mainly the United States of America and Europe. The severe contagious nature of COVID-19 has developed an unprecedented and unpredictable situation in the world [2].

The world's current population is 7.6 billion in 2020 [4], and approximately half of the world's population (3.9 billion people) are currently facing lockdown and quarantine measures in their homes [5]. However, despite the safety measures, the transmission of the disease and its subsequent mortalities have continued [6]. A year later, in February 2021, there is still no availability of a specific recommended drug therapy to treat SARS-CoV patients. However, Pfizer/BioNTech, Moderna, and a few other recommended vaccines have recently become available and are being used to contain the virus. These vaccines have been advised to people 16 years of age and older, and they provide immunogenicity for at least 119 days after the first vaccination.

Some meteorological factors are involved in the transmission and magnitude of the spread of viruses [7, 8]. More recently, a few published studies demonstrated that these factors include respiratory droplets of various sizes [9], warm weather, and humidity [10]. These factors are involved in the coronavirus's further spreading, which has already infected over 110 million people worldwide [3]. Despite recent efforts to understand the epidemiological trends of a novel coronavirus, the science community, researchers, policymakers, and the general population search for more information about the transmission and current biological and epidemiological situation [1] and its association with weather conditions, including heat and humidity.

Transmission of COVID-19

The first case of SARS-CoV-2 appeared in the last week of December 2019, amongst people living in and visiting Wuhan, China [3]. COVID-19 initially originated from bats, and seafood and has an "animal to animal, animal to human, and human to human" transmission [Figure 2.1] [6].

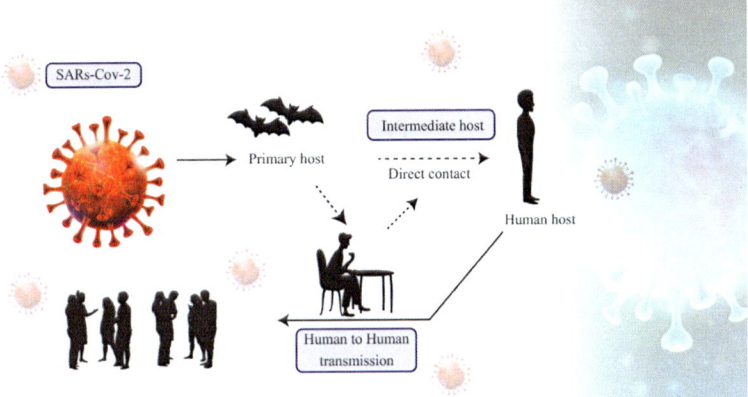

Figure 2.1: Spread of SARS-COV-2.

The primary sources of transmission from human to human are airborne and respiratory droplets. Humans produce respiratory droplets of 0.1 to 1000 μm in size. The transmission can be variable based on the droplet size, environment, inertia, gravity, evaporation, and how far emitted droplets and aerosols can travel and stay in the environment. The transmission is also based on the place, weather, and interaction, such as communication, laughing, coughing, or sneezing. The literature shows that droplets with a size of about ~100 μm produced during coughing and sneezing rapidly underwent gravitational settling. These droplets of 100-μm will settle to the ground from 8 feet in 4.6 s, whereas a 1-μm aerosol particle will take about 12 hours to settle in the environment [9]. The current evidence suggests that SARS-CoV-2 infection spreads from human to human directly, or indirectly, via contaminated objects or surfaces or close contact with infected people, via oral or nasal secretions. These include saliva and respiratory secretions, etc. [Figure 2.2].

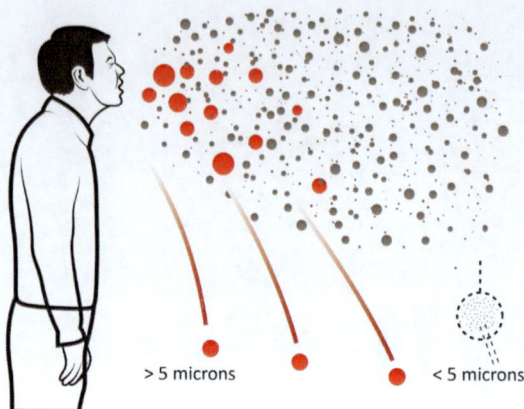

Figure 2.2: The droplet and airborne transmission of SARS-CoV-2 infection during coughing and sneezing.

People worldwide are highly anxious about the contagious nature of the disease and the pandemic calamities. This, for the first time, has developed a volatile and threatening situation throughout all nations. The transmission of the coronavirus, and its subsequent incidence and mortalities, has continued worldwide. However, there is a great debate on meteorological factors concerning the transmission and magnitude of the spread of viruses [10]. It may be less prevalent in countries closer to the equator, where heat and humidity increase. The science community has conducted a few studies on the weather changes and COVID-19 pandemic in the various regions of the globe where temperature and humidity has been swiftly changing.

The COVID-19 pandemic in the world's top ten hottest and top ten coldest countries

The weather allied conditions impact the air, water, soil, food, ecosystem, feelings, behaviors, and patterns of health and disease [10]. Worldwide, many countries have extreme temperatures and humidity. Meo et al., 2020 [11] conducted a study on the world's top ten hottest and top ten coldest countries and their association with temperature, humidity, and the COVID-19 pandemic. The selection of the countries was based on the daily mean temperature from the date of appearance of the initial cases of COVID-19, December 29, 2019, to May 12, 2020. In the world's ten hottest countries, the mean temperature was 26.31 ± 1.51^0C and humidity $44.67\pm4.97\%$. However, in the world's ten coldest countries, the mean temperature was 6.19 ± 1.61^0C and humidity $57.26\pm2.35\%$ [Table 2.1]. The data on the global outbreak of COVID-19, new daily cases, and deaths were recorded from the World Health Organization [3], and daily information on temperature and humidity was obtained from the metrological web "Time and Date" [12]. The population of these countries was obtained from the World Bank, 2020 [4]. In the ten warmest countries, the combined mean population was 192035178±131644730.8, and in the coldest countries, the mean population was 62753407± 36653385.06. In the warmest countries, the mean temperature was 26.31±1.51^{0}C, and humidity was 44.67±4.97%. However, in the coldest countries, the mean temperature was 6.19±1.61^{0}C, and moisture was 57.26±2.35% (Table 2.1).

Table 2.1: Comparison of temperature and humidity between the world's top ten hottest countries compared to the world's top ten coldest countries

World's Top Ten Hottest Countries			World's Top Ten Coldest Countries		
Country	Temperature	Humidity	Country	Temperature	Humidity
Iran	16.28	38.76	Finland	-1.56	66.41
Algeria	22.50	68.69	Canada	1.71	61.43
Pakistan	22.60	54.44	Norway	2.12	56.34
India	28.91	47.25	Belarus	3.54	57.96
Mexico	24.63	26.37	Russian Federation	5.76	60.82
Kuwait	28.30	32.32	Estonia	5.80	62.58
United Arab Emirates	28.74	39.96	Sweden	6.76	59.97
Saudi Arabia	29.39	21.39	Kazakhstan	10.55	55.05
Oman	29.42	53.37	United States of America	12.86	52.68
Ghana	32.37	64.18	Austria	14.35	39.33
Mean ± SEM	26.31±1.51	44.67±4.97	**Mean ± SEM**	6.19 ± 1.61	57.26±2.35

Temperature and humidity were recorded from the Date of initial cases that appeared from December 29 to May 12, 2020. Daily cases and daily deaths were recorded from December 29 to May 12, 2020. Data presented in Mean and SEM. [Table adopted after permission from author and publisher] [11].

Meo et al., 2020 [11] further reported that in countries with higher temperatures, the mean daily cases, cumulative cases, daily deaths, and cumulative deaths were significantly lower in comparison to countries with lower temperatures. The authors further analyzed that the COVID-19 cases per one million people in countries with high temperatures were 711.23 and mean daily deaths were 16.27 compared to countries with low temperatures where COVID-19 cases per million people were 1685.99 and deaths were 86.40. The number of patients and fatalities per one million people was significantly lower in countries with high temperatures than countries with low temperatures [Figure 2.3].

Table 2.2: Comparison of incidence and mortality of daily cases, cumulative cases, daily deaths, and cumulative deaths between the world's top ten hottest countries compared to the world's top ten coldest countries

Parameters	Countries with high temperature (n=10)	Countries with low temperature (n=10)	Significance Level
Daily Cases	407.12±24.33	1876.72±207.37	0.008
Cumulative Cases	9094.34±708.29	44232.38±5875.11	0.02
Daily Deaths	17.80±1.35	100.41±14.88	0.442
Cumulative Deaths	452.84±43.30	2008.29±310.13	0.001

Temperature and humidity were recorded from the Date of initial cases from December 29 to May 12, 2020.

Daily cases and daily deaths were recorded from December 29 to May 12, 2020. Data presented in Mean and SEM.

[Table adopted after permission from author and publisher] [11].

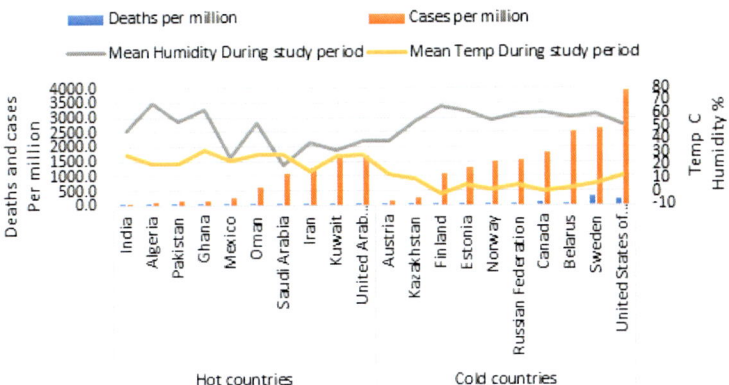

Figure 2.3: Daily cases and daily deaths per one million population in the world's top ten hottest and coldest countries. [Figure adopted after permission obtained from the author and publisher] [11].

The impact of temperature and humidity on the epidemiological trends on the number of cases and deaths and correlation coefficient values are presented in Table 2.3. The results revealed a significant negative correlation between the number of new daily cases and deaths in countries with high temperatures and low humidity (warmest countries), compared to those countries with low temperatures and high humidity (coldest countries) (Table 2.3).

Table 2.3. The correlation coefficient between daily cases, cumulative cases, daily deaths, and cumulative deaths between the world's top ten hottest countries compared to the world's top ten coldest countries

Comparable parameters	Correlation Coefficient in countries with high temperature (n=10)	Significance Level	Correlation Coefficient in countries with low temperature (n=10)	Significance Level
Temperature-Daily Cases	-0.016	p=0.002	0.338	p=0.001
Temperature-Cumulative Cases	-0.115	p=0.001	0.302	p=0.001
Temperature-Daily Deaths	-0.248	p=0.001	0.282	p=0.001

Temperature-Cumulative Deaths	-0.241	p=0.001	0.302	p=0.001
Humidity-Daily Cases	-0.166	p=0.001	-0.082	p=0.013
Humidity-Cumulative Cases	-0.145	p=0.001	-0.089	p=0.007
Humidity-Daily Deaths	-0.104	p=0.003	-0.078	p=0.019
Humidity-Cumulative Deaths	-0.103	p=0.003	-0.078	p=0.019

Temperature and humidity were recorded from the Date of initial cases from December 29 to May 12, 2020.

Correlation coefficient based on daily cases and daily deaths recorded from December 29 to May 12, 2020. [Table adopted after permission from author and publisher] [11].

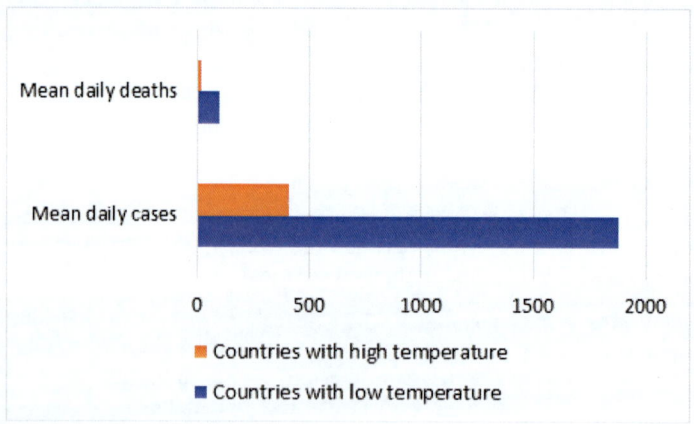

Figure 2.4: Mean daily cases and daily deaths in the world's top ten hottest countries and coldest countries.

[Figure adopted after permission obtained from the author and publisher] [11].

While a large number of studies have been published on the COVID-19 pandemic [13], limited research has been conducted on the correlation of this pandemic and its association with weather conditions. Chan et al., 2011

[14] demonstrated that the SARS-CoV-2 virus has better stability at low temperature and in low humidity environments; hence, it may facilitate the transmission of the disease. The authors reported that the coronavirus's viability was rapidly lost at higher temperatures and higher relative humidity. Wu et al., 2020 [15] assessed the impact of temperature and relative humidity on new daily cases and new daily deaths of COVID-19. The authors identified that temperature and relative humidity negatively affect new daily cases and new deaths.

Qi et al., 2020 [16] found that temperature and humidity significantly negatively correlated with COVID-19. Their study findings suggest that daily temperature and relative humidity influenced the occurrence of COVID-19. However, the association between COVID-19 and temperature and humidity was not consistent throughout Mainland China. Meo et al., 2020 [11] study results revealed that countries with high temperatures and low humidity levels were associated with a decreased number of daily cases and deaths caused by COVID-19. The results showed a significant negative correlation between the decrease in new daily cases and deaths in countries with high temperature and low humidity (warmest countries) than those with low temperature and high humidity levels (coldest countries). The results reflect that high temperature and low moisture work better to minimize new daily cases and deaths.

On the contrary, Xie and Zhu et al., 2020 [17] examined the correlation between COVID-19 and temperature in China. Their results showed a positive linear association between the number of COVID-19 cases and the mean temperature. They did not find any evidence supporting the hypothesis that COVID-19 patients could decline when the weather becomes warmer. In another study, Ma and colleagues, 2020 [18] reported an increase in diurnal temperature associated with increased COVID-19 deaths. However, an increase in humidity was related to a decrease in the deaths caused by COVID-19. Wang et al., 2020 [19] investigated the association of temperature on the spread of COVID-19 and claimed that temperature significantly affects the transmission of COVID-19. Bannister-Tyrrell et al., 2020 [20] demonstrated that an average temperature increase was negatively correlated with the number of SARS-CoV-2 cases. In addition to these facts and figures, we further highlighted the various regions in which there is a significant fluctuation in the temperature and humidity and its linkage with SARS-CoV-2 cases and deaths.

Weather Conditions and the COVID-19 pandemic in the Middle East

The Middle East region comprises 17 countries with a population of about 371 million people [4]. This region has relatively high temperatures, homogenous Arab ethnicity, and the same socioeconomic culture. The rapid changes in the socioeconomic conditions have caused swift urbanization and variations in socioeconomic and environmental conditions in the Middle East. The COVID-19 pandemic also highly affected this part of the world. Meo et al., 2020 [10] selected all the six "Gulf Cooperation Council (GCC) countries, of the Middle East region including Saudi Arabia, the United Arab Emirates, Bahrain, Kuwait, Qatar, and Oman." Meo et al. [10] analyzed the impact of temperature and humidity on the daily new cases and deaths due to COVID-19 in all six GCC countries. The daily mean temperature and humidity were recorded from the date of appearance of the first case of COVID-19 in the GCC region, from January 29, 2020, to May 15, 2020. The mean temperature and humidity in Oman were 29.89±0.48, 51.32±2.21; the United Arab Emirates 29.03±0.55, 39.45±1.58; Kuwait 28.85±0.52, 31.16±1.68; Bahrain 27.99±0.49, 44.87±1.78; Saudi Arabia 29.75±0.55, 20.59±1.12 and Qatar 29.67±0.55, 40.29±2.04. The overall mean temperature in all these six GCC countries was 29.20 ±0.30°C, and humidity was 37.95 ±4.40% (Figures 2.5 and 2.6).

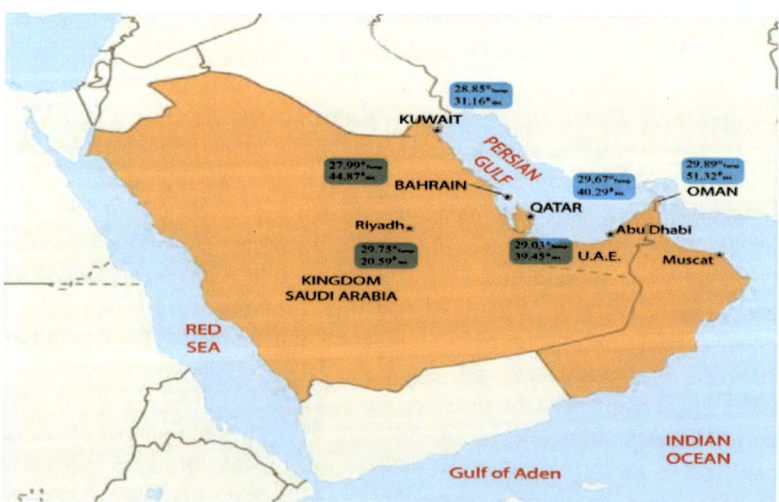

Figure 2.5: Mean temperature and humidity in the GCC region of the Middle East. [Figure adopted after permission from the author and publisher] [10].

In GCC countries, an increase in humidity was associated with a decrease in the number of daily cases and deaths from COVID-19. However, an increase in temperature was also associated with an increase in the number of daily cases and daily deaths due to COVID-19. Meo et al., [10] further demonstrated that the daily growth factor for patients and deaths in GCC countries shows a declining trend. The association between COVID-19, temperature, and humidity was not consistent throughout the GCC region in the Middle East. However, the climate is swiftly changing in the region, and further studies may be conducted during the peak of the summer season to reach better and more precise conclusions.

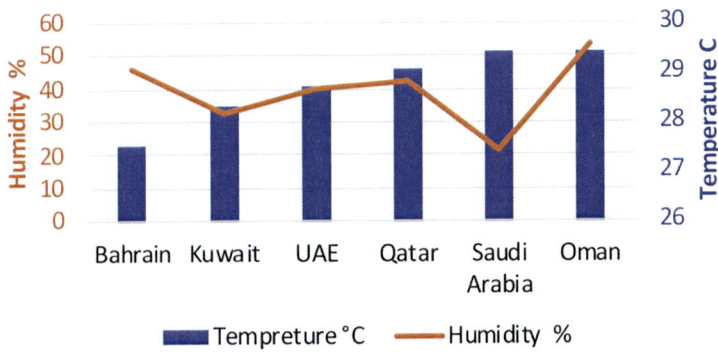

Figure 2.6: Temperature and humidity in GCC countries. [Figure adopted after permission from author and publisher] [10].

Weather conditions and the COVID-19 pandemic in European countries

Europe is the sixth-largest continent, situated in the Northern Hemisphere and mostly in the Eastern Hemisphere. There are 50 states in Europe, with 747 million people, about 11% of the world population [21, 22]. From 50 European states, Meo et al., 2020 [23] randomly selected 10 European countries, including Russia, the United Kingdom, Spain, Italy, Germany, Turkey, France, Belgium, the Netherlands, and Belarus. The European region has relatively homogenous weather conditions, ethnicity, socioeconomic culture, and health care system. The daily new cases and deaths due to COVID-19 and the daily information on meteorological conditions, temperature, and humidity were recorded from the date of appearance of the first case of SARS-CoV-2 in the European region, January 27, 2020, to July 17, 2020. The daily mean temperature during this period was 17.07±**0.18**0C, and humidity was 54.78±0.47%.

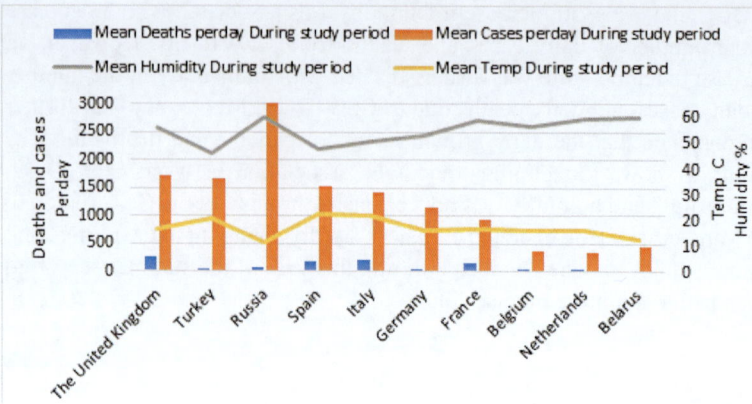

Figure 2.7: Mean temperature, humidity, number of daily cases, and daily deaths due to the COVID-19 pandemic in European countries. [Adopted after permission obtained from the author and publisher] [23].

Meo et al., 2020 [23] explored the impact of heat and humidity on the incidence and mortality rates due to the COVID-19 pandemic in 10 European countries to understand the dispersal pattern of the COVID-19 pandemic. The epidemiologic and public health facts considering the periodic variation in weather conditions are essential factors in defining the seasonal behavior of some forms of diseases and health phenomena. The authors identified that an increase in relative humidity was associated with a decrease in the number of daily cases and deaths. However, a temperature rise was allied with an upsurge in the number of daily cases and deaths due to the COVID-19 pandemic in European countries. The change in weather conditions is believed to alter the ecosystem pattern at broad regional levels [24]. The impact of weather events is traumatic, leading to injuries, lethal diseases, and deaths. Extreme weather events include heatwaves, cold spells, heavy rain, and snowfalls, etc. These weather conditions have a significant influence on the pattern of health and disease [25].

Table 2.4. Temperature, humidity, number of daily cases, cumulative cases, daily deaths, and cumulative deaths due to the COVID-19 pandemic in European countries.

Countries	Temperature 0C (Mean ± SEM)	Humidity % (Mean ± SEM)	Daily Cases (Mean ± SEM)	Cumulative Cases (Mean ± SEM)	Daily Deaths (Mean ± SEM)	Cumulative Deaths (Mean ± SEM)
Russia	11.58±0.73	59.79±1.55	4492.33±316.73	221994.73±20133.13	71.73±5.61	2910.13±292.70
United Kingdom	16.56±0.44	55.97±1.41	1737.31±239.34	141853.67±9701.21	266.97±32.60	20242.77±1421.50
Spain	22.73±0.59	47.32±1.52	1535.30±172.25	144515.35±8162.83	195.56±23.80	16076.84±947.54
Italy	21.69±0.46	50.35±1.17	1425.35±134.00	140949.22±7634.66	204.77±19.11	19454.39±1114.02
Germany	15.77±0.50	52.94±1.49	1167.69±125.26	107958.17±6239.47	52.80±5.89	4435.39±298.82
Turkey	20.85±0.59	46.08±1.55	1668.25±107.41	120192.20±6380.17	41.84±3.14	3151.66±171.75
France	16.56±0.43	58.57±1.32	938.80±103.17	84509.58±5039.22	170.63±22.95	15398.05±995.18
Belgium	15.84±0.44	57.18±1.43	381.13±38.99	33812.28±2032.35	59.02±7.56	5190.72±336.21
Netherlands	16.07±0.42	59.45±1.33	361.23±31.78	32203.95±1590.58	43.15±4.61	3892.99±206.07
Belarus	13.00±0.63	59.59±1.66	465.41±40.48	26236.71±2102.62	3.44±0.24	161.52±13.27
Mean ± SEM	17.07±0.18	54.78±0.47	14445.61±59.34	107814.61±3192.75	116.09±5.87	9520.72±309.06

Data presented from the Date of appearance of the first case of SARS-COV-2 in European countries, January 27, 2020, to July 17, 2020. Values are presented in Mean and SEM. Temperature °C: Humidity%. [Table adopted after permission obtained from the author and publisher] [23].

Harmooshi et al., 2020 [26[reported the environmental conditions necessary for the survival and spread of the SARS-CoV-2 infection. SARS-CoV-2 is sensitive to humidity; lifespan at 50% humidity is more extended than at 30%. The virus may tolerate about nine days at 25°C, but the lifespan may reduce if the temperature rises to 30°C. The authors further reported that low temperature, and a dry and unventilated environment may affect the stability and spread of the virus.

Sajadi et al., 2020 [27] conducted a study on the COVID-19 pandemic and temperature and humidity; they did not find an association between weather changes and the spread of SARS-CoV-2. Similarly, Huang et al. [28] study results demonstrate an optimal climatic zone in which SARS-CoV-2 increases in an ambient environment. The findings demonstrate that the COVID-19 pandemic may episodically appear, and outbreaks may recur in metropolitan areas in the autumn season.

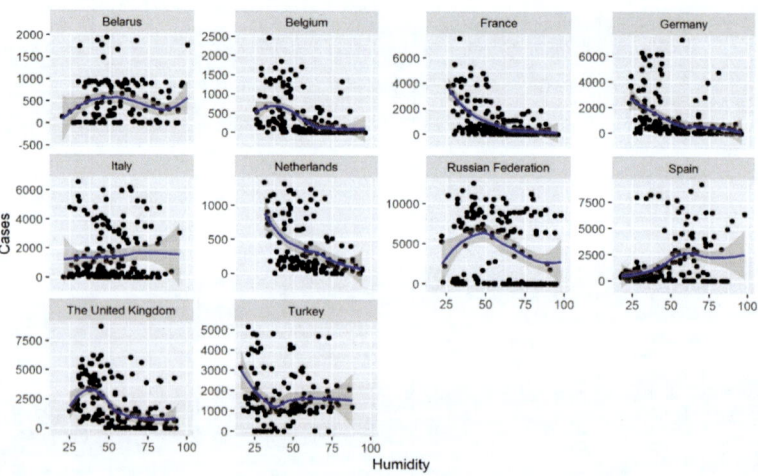

Figure 2.8: The trend of humidity and daily cases due to the COVID-19 pandemic in European countries.

[Figure adopted after permission obtained from the author and publisher] [23].

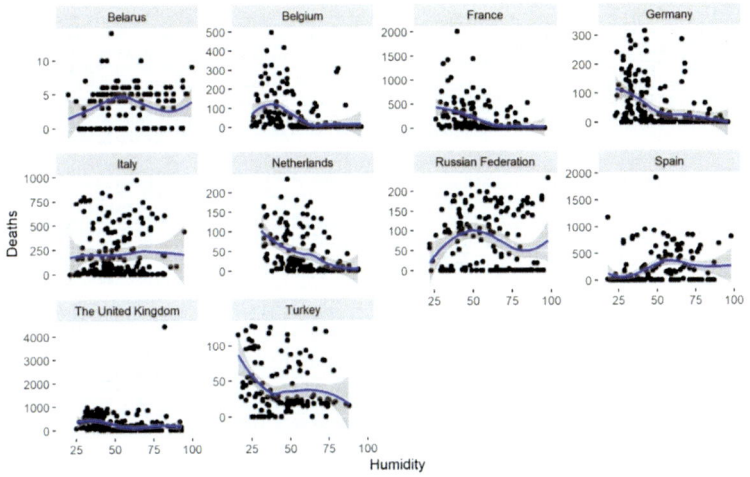

Figure 2.9: The trend of humidity and daily deaths due to the COVID-19 pandemic in European countries.

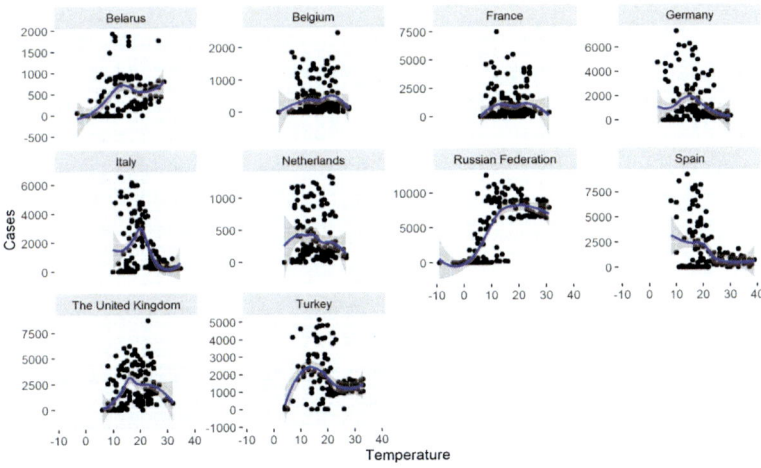

Figure 2.10: The trend of temperature and number of daily cases due to the COVID-19 pandemic in European countries. [Figure adopted after permission obtained from the author and publisher] [23].

[Figure adopted after permission obtained from the author and publisher] [23].

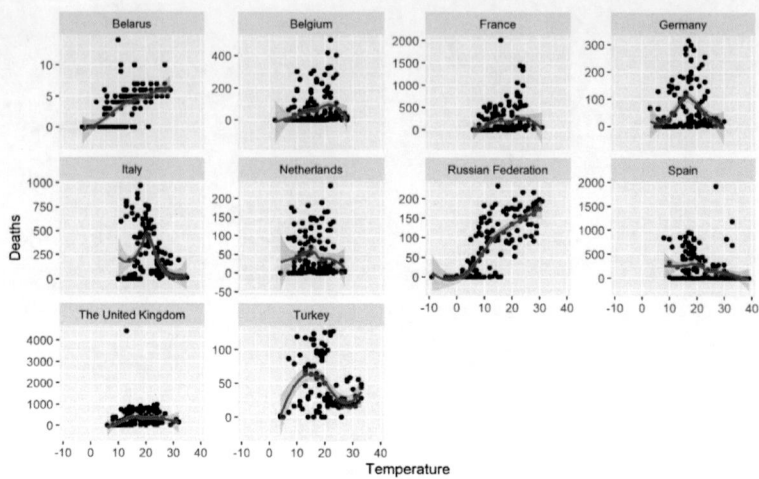

Figure 2.11: The trend of temperature and daily deaths due to the COVID-19 pandemic in European countries.

[Figure adopted after permission obtained from the author and publisher] [23].

In the human body, each cell is very vital and plays a significant role in controlling various body functions. The human body needs its normal biological, physiological, and environmental conditions to perform and maintain different body functions. The meteorological conditions, including temperature and humidity, are essential to maintain normal body functions. The change in the environment can change the pattern of health and disease [21].

Extreme temperatures, either very cold or very hot, are not physiologically suitable for normal body functions. The respiratory system is highly vulnerable to pollution and microorganisms. In cold weather, the relative risk of respiratory disease increases, and exposure to low temperatures can impair immune mechanisms [29-31]. It is a fact that respiratory infections are more frequent during cold and low humidity conditions [32]. Evidence from earlier studies has documented that viruses are more stable in cold and dry conditions, as low temperatures facilitate ideal conditions for virus attachment, replication, and transmission [33, 34]. The exact mechanism of the interaction of the novel coronavirus is still unclear. However, the probable reason may be that a combination of low temperature and humidity makes the respiratory mucosa more prone to rupture and creates opportunities for virus invasion [35].

Conclusions

The present chapter findings revealed a decrease in new daily cases and deaths in countries with high temperatures than those with low temperatures. The COVID-19 cases and deaths per million population were significantly lower in countries with higher temperatures than countries with lower temperatures. Similarly, in European countries, an increase in relative humidity was allied with a decrease in the number of daily cases and deaths due to the COVID-19 pandemic. These findings have outcomes for policymakers, health officials, and the public about the impact of temperature and humidity on the epidemiological trends of COVID-19. Essential measures must be taken to control the source of SARS-CoV-2 infection and transmission to prevent the pandemic from spreading further, both at regional and international levels. More attention should be paid to regions that endure low temperatures as this environment is more suitable for the viability of the novel coronavirus SARS-CoV-2, the COVID-19 pandemic.

References

1. Meo SA, Al-Khlaiwi T, Usmani AM, Meo AS, Klonoff DC, Hoang TD. Biological and Epidemiological Trends in the Prevalence and Mortality due to Outbreaks of Novel Coronavirus COVID-19. J King Saud Univ Sci, 2020; 32: 2495-2499. doi: 10.1016/j.jksus.2020.04.004.

2. Meo SA, Alhowikan AM, Al-Khlaiwi T, Meo IM, Halepoto DM, Iqbal M, Usmani AM, Hajjar W, Ahmed N. Novel coronavirus 2019-nCoV: prevalence, biological and clinical characteristics comparison with SARS-CoV and MERS-CoV. Eur Rev Med Pharmacol Sci. 2020. 24: 2012-2019.

3. World Health Organization: Coronavirus. Available at: https://www.who.int/health-topics/coronavirus. Cited Date June 24, 2020.

4. World Bank. Population total. Available at: https:// data.worldbank.org/ indicator/sp.pop.totl. Cited Date. July 12, 2020.

5. Daily Mail. 3.9 billion people are currently called on to stay in their homes. Available at: https://www. dailymail.co.uk/news/article-8181001/3-9-billion- people-currently-called-stay-homes-coronavirus.html.

6. Shereen MA, Khan S, Kazmi A, Bashir N, Siddique R. COVID-19 infection: Origin, transmission, and characteristics of human coronaviruses. J Adv Res. 2020; (24): 91-98. doi: 10.1016/j.jare.2020.03.005.

7. Şahin M. Impact of weather on COVID-19 pandemic in Turkey. Sci Total Environ 2020; 728: 138810.

8. Nassar MS, Bak hrebah MA, Meo SA, Alsua beyl MS, Zaher WA. Global seasonal occurrence of middle east respiratory syndrome coronavirus (MERS-CoV) infection. Eur Rev Med Pharmacol Sci 2018; 22: 3913-3918.

9. Prather KA, Wang CC, Schooley RT. Reducing the transmission of SARS-CoV-2. Science. 2020 June 26;368(6498):1422-1424. doi: 10.1126/science.abc6197.

10. Meo SA, Abukhalaf AA, Alomar AA, Alsalame NM, Al-Khlaiwi T, Usmani AM. Effect of temperature and humidity on the dynamics of daily new cases and deaths due to COVID-19 outbreak in Gulf countries in Middle East Region. Eur Rev Med Pharmacol Sci. 2020 Jul;24(13):7524-7533. doi: 10.26355/eurrev_202007_21927.

11. Meo SA, Abukhalaf AA, Alomar AA, I.Z. AL-beeshi, Alhowikan A.Climate, and COVID-19 pandemic: effect of heat and humidity on the incidence and mortality in world's top ten hottest and top ten coldest countries. European Review for Medical and Pharmacological Sciences, 2020; 24: 8232-8238.

12. Time and Date, weather: Available at https://www.timeanddate.com/weather/saudi-arabia/riyadh/historic?month=2&year=2020. Cited Date May 20, 2020.

13. Spiteri G, Fielding J, Diercke M, Campese C, Enouf V, Gaymard A, Bella A, Sognamiglio P. First cases of coronavirus disease 2019 (COVID-19) in the WHO European Region, January 24 to February 21 2020. Euro Surveill. 2020; 25: 2000178. doi: 10.2807/1560-7917. ES.2020.25.9.2000178.

14. Chan, KH, Peiris JS, Lam SY, Poon LL, Yuen KY, Seto WH. The Effects of Temperature and Relative Humidity on the Viability of the SARS Coronavirus. Adv Virol, 2011; 2011: 734690. doi: 10.1155/2011/734690.

15. Wu Y, Jin W, Liu J, Ma Q, Yuan J, Wang Y. Effects of temperature and humidity on the daily new cases and new deaths of COVID-19 in 166 countries. Sci. Total. Environ. 2020. 729: 139051. doi: 10.1016/j.scitotenv.2020.139051.

16. Qi H, Xiao S, Shi R, Ward MP, Chen Y, Tu W, Su Q, Wang W, Wang X, Zhang Z. COVID-19 transmission in Mainland China is associated with temperature and humidity: A time-series analysis. Sci Total Environ. 2020 August 1;728:138778. doi: 10.1016/j.scitotenv.2020.138778.

17. Xie J, Zhu Y. Association between ambient temperature and COVID-19 infection in 122 cities from China. Sci Total Environ. 2020. 724. doi: 10.1016/j.scitotenv.2020.138201

18. Ma Y, Zhao Y, Liu J, He X, Wang B, Fu S. Effects of temperature variation and humidity on the death of COVID-19 in Wuhan, China. Sci Total Environ. 2020; 724: doi: 10.1016/j.scitotenv.2020.138226

19. Wang M, Jiang A, Gong L, Luo L, Guo W, Li C, Zheng J, Li C, Yang B, Zeng J, Chen Y, Zheng K, Li H. Temperature significant change COVID-19 transmission in 429 cities. medRxiv. 2020; doi: 10.1101/2020.02.22.20025791.

20. Bannister-Tyrrell M, Meyer A, Faverjon C, Cameron A. Preliminary evidence that higher temperatures are associated with lower incidence of COVID-19, for cases reported globally up to February 29 2020. MedRxiv. 2020. doi: 10.1101/2020.03.18.20036731.

21. World Population Prospects: The 2019 Revision" population.un.org. United Nations Department of Economic and Social Affairs, Population Division. Cited Date, June 24, 2020.

22. Worldometer. Available at: https://www.worldometers.info/demographics/demographics-of-europe/ Cited date July 12, 2002.

23. Meo SA, Abukhalaf AA, Alomar A, Sumaya OY, Sami W, Shafi KM, Meo AS, Usmani AM, Akram J. Effect of Heat and Humidity on the Incidence and Mortality due to COVID-19 Pandemic in European Countries. Eur Rev Med Pharmacol Sci. 2020. 24: (16):

24. Ballester F, Michelozzi P, Iñiguez C. Weather, climate, and public health. J Epidemiol Community Health. 2003; 57: 759-60. doi: 10.1136/jech.57.10.75 PMID: 14573565

25. Meo SA. Lung Functions in Health and Disease: Basics and applied with MCQs. King Saud University Press, 2019; pp 1-12. ISBN: 978-603-507-610-4.

26. Harmooshi NN, Shirbandi K, Rahim F. Environmental concern regarding the effect of humidity and temperature on 2019-nCoV survival: fact or fiction. Environ Sci Pollut Res Int. 2020 26: 110.doi: 10.1007/s11356-020-09733-w

27. Sajadi MM, Habibzadeh P, Vintzileos A, Shokouhi S, Miralles-Wilhelm F, Amoroso A (2020b) Temperature and latitude analysis to predict potential spread and seasonality for COVID-19. JAMA Net Open. 2020; 3: e2011834. doi: 10.1001/jamanetworkopen.2020.11834.

28. Huang Z, Huang J, Qianqing Gu, Pengyue Du, Liang H, Dong Q. Optimal temperature zone for the dispersal of COVID-19. Sci Total Environ 2020; 736: 139487.

29. Shephard RJ, Shek PN. Cold exposure and immune function Can. J. Physiol. Pharmacol. 1998; 76 (9) 828-836.

30. Castellani JWM, Brenner IK, Rhind SG. Cold exposure: human immune responses and intracellular cytokine expression. Med Sci Sports Exerc. 2020; 34 (12): 2013-20.

31. Luo B, Liu J, Fei G, Han T, Zhang K, Wang L, Shi H, Zhang L, Ruan Y, Niu J. Impact of probable interaction of low temperature and ambient fine particulate matter on the function of rats alveolar macrophages. Environ. Toxicol. Pharmacol. 2017; 49: 172-178, Doi: 10.1016/j.etap.2016.12.011.

32. Davis RE, McGregor GR, Enfield KB. Humidity: a review and primer on atmospheric moisture and human health. Environ. Res. 2016; 144: 106-116.

33. Lin K, Fong D, Zhu B, Karlberg J. Environmental factors on the SARS epidemic: air temperature, the passage of time and multiplicative effect of hospital infection. Epidemiol. Infect. 2006; 134, 223-230.

34. Casanova LM, Jeonm S, Rutalam WA, Weber DJ, Sobsey MD. Effects of air temperature and relative humidity on coronavirus survival on surfaces. Appl. Environ. Microbiol. 2010; 76: 2712-2717.

35. Zhou ZX, Jiang CQ. Effect of environment and occupational hygiene factors of hospital infection on SARS outbreak. Zhonghua lao dong wei sheng zhi ye bing za zhi, 2004; 22: 261-263.

Environmental Pollution and the COVID-19 Pandemic

Chapter 03

Sultan Ayoub Meo

Abstract

The Severe Acute Respiratory Syndrome-2 (SARS-CoV-2) infection, also known as the COVID-19 pandemic, transmits from animal to animal, animal to human, and human to human through droplets, via direct or indirect contact. During the past two decades, there has been a tremendous shift in social demographics; people are shifting from rural to urban regions resulting in an upward change in the urban population. This rapid, unplanned urbanization and industrialization has contributed to environmental pollution. Urbanization and industrialization are the key contributing factors to the ongoing change in global climate, with increasingly poor air quality and environmental pollution. Particulate matter, carbon monoxide, nitrogen dioxide, sulfur dioxide, ozone, volatile organic compounds (VOCs), and polycyclic aromatic hydrocarbons (PAHs) are major air pollutants and have become a leading cause of innumerable illnesses. People are residing in regions with long-term exposure to polluted air, leading to chronic respiratory and coronary artery diseases. The literature supports an association between environmental pollutants and human respiratory viruses, interacting to adversely affect the respiratory and other body organs. The global science literature established an association between increased environmental pollutants and rising cases and deaths due to SARS-CoV-2 infection. It is essential to take severe preventive measures to decrease ecological contaminants. This would be potentially beneficial to reduce the risk of exposure to, and subsequent transmission of, the SARS-CoV-2 infection, and fight against the COVID-19 pandemic.

Keywords: Environmental pollution, SARS-CoV-2, COVID-19 pandemic

Introduction

Over the past three decades, environmental pollution has been an emerging global health problem [1]. Swift urbanization and industrialization have increased ecological pollution to a dangerous level. The various sources of pollution change the arrangement and composition of the environment, including air, water, and soil [1]. Environmental pollution is the contagion of the biological, chemical, and physical elements which adversely affect the everyday environment. It is an unfavorable change due to direct or indirect human-associated activities [2].

Environmental pollutants may be "dust, gases, fumes, geochemical substances, biological organisms, chemicals, toxic metals, radionuclides, physical substances, heat, radiation and sound waves" [2]. The undesirable effects of these pollutants directly or indirectly affect human beings via organisms or the climate. Based on the pollutants' biological, physical, and chemical nature, environmental pollution is categorized into various types: air, water, soil, noise, radioactive, and thermal. All these types of pollution damage the ecosystem and are a source of numerous health hazards [2].

Data revealed by the World Health Organization (WHO) indicates that air pollution levels remain at dangerously high levels in many parts of the world. More than 80% of people live in urban areas, 91% of the world's population live in regions where air quality exceeds WHO guideline limits and 9 out of 10 people breathe air containing high levels of pollutants. Every year, environmental risks such as indoor and outdoor air pollution, second-hand smoke, unsafe water, lack of sanitation, and inadequate hygiene take the lives of 1.7 million children under the age of 5 years [3]. Moreover, 1 in 4 deaths of children under five years of age is due to an unhealthy polluted environment.

There are about 4.2 million deaths every year due to exposure to ambient outdoor air pollution and 3.8 million deaths due to household exposure to smoke from various daily life activities. Air pollution causes 2.4 million deaths due to cardiovascular diseases, 1.8 million deaths due to respiratory illnesses, and 1.4 million deaths due to cerebrovascular accidents (stroke) per annum. It has also been reported that 24% of all stroke deaths, 25% of heart disease deaths, and 43% of all lung disease and lung cancer deaths are potentially due to environmental pollution [3].

There has been a tremendous shift in social demographics, and people are shifting from rural to urban regions to reside in metropolitan cities, mainly. This rapid migration causes various health hazards in urban areas due to the increase in the population. Environmental pollution has been a major health hazard for the general population. The respiratory system is highly vulnerable to environmental pollution. Respiratory viruses are a leading cause of severe respiratory infections and affect other body organs and systems. These viruses are a challenging issue of great importance. "Particulate matter (PM), carbon monoxide, sulfur dioxide, nitrogen oxides, ozone, volatile organic compounds (VOCs) and polycyclic aromatic hydrocarbons

(PAHs)" are major air pollutants that are the main cause of innumerable illnesses. The literature supports an association between environmental pollutants and human respiratory viruses interacting to adversely affect the respiratory and cardiovascular systems and other body organs [4].

Presently, the entire world faces the devastating impact, and the challenges, posed by the Severe Acute Respiratory Syndrome-2 (SARS-CoV-2) infection, also known as the COVID-19 pandemic. The swift spread of this novel coronavirus from person to person is through the "direct or indirect contact with an infected subject, respiratory droplets emitted through coughing and sneezing that can reach an uninfected subject, and inhalation of small airborne particles remaining in the air" [5-7]. The swift spread of the SARS-CoV-2 infection has led the entire world into a hostile and unstable situation.

The various climate and environmental pollution factors directly impact coronavirus diffusion [8-10]. Thus, it supports the fact that urban areas with higher environmental pollution had higher infection rates and deaths due to exceedingly high levels of particulate matter or ozone levels. The science community strongly believes that air pollution is one of the determining indicators affecting the spread of COVID-19 [11]. Furthermore, geographical, demographic, environmental, and climatological factors influence infectious diseases, especially in urban areas.

Worldwide, the science community has established a link between various environmental pollutants and the increasing number of SARS-CoV-2 cases and deaths. Morawska and Cao (2020) [12] reported that air is the main transmission route of SARS-CoV-2 infection. Together with specific climatic conditions supporting the viral particles that remain in the air, environmental pollutants could promote the indirect diffusion of SARS-CoV-2. In another study, Coccia (2020) [10, 11] demonstrated the dynamics of COVID-19, which spread due to air pollution-to-human transmission. The findings of the studies suggest a strong association between environmental pollution and SARS-CoV-2 infection.

Environmental Pollution and Influenza

In recent years, many studies have been published in leading science journals that have established a risk factor relationship between environmental pollution and adverse respiratory and cardiovascular health outcomes. Exposure to environmental pollutants can cause oxidative stress, resulting in the production of free radicals. This, in turn, may damage the respiratory system, impairing the resistance to viral and bacterial infections [13].

Pothirat et al. (2019) [14] determined the relationship between daily environmental pollutants and emergency hospitalization visits for severe respiratory, cardiovascular, and cerebrovascular disease. The authors found that environmental pollutants were allied to high mortality among hospitalized patients and community residents. It shows that environmental pollution is a leading cause of various cardio-respiratory diseases and deaths.

Su et al. (2019) [15] computed the short-term effects of air pollutants, "PM2.5, PM10, O_3, CO, SO_2, and NO_2". It was identified that subjects from different age groups were susceptible to environmental pollutants including PM2.5, PM10, and CO. Air pollutants, mainly "PM2.5, PM10, CO, and SO_2," can increase the risk of influenza-like illness. Similarly, Chen et al. (2018) [16] established a causal connection between environmental pollution and human influenza cases. In another study, Chen et al. (2017) [17] identified that ecological pollutants and particulate matter (PM2.5) could cause 10.7% of influenza cases and increase the risk of influenza, especially in winter weather. In addition to meteorological factors, "air pollutants including particulate matter PM2.5, carbon monoxide, ozone, sulfur dioxide, nitrogen dioxide and haze are among the frequent environmental pollutants which may affect influenza transmission" [18,19]. Zhao et al. (2016) [20] identified that short-term exposure to PM2.5 might involve air pollution-induced immune disorders and diseases. Once immunity is impaired, it can cause various debilitating health problems. In this section, we reviewed the scientific literature that shows an association between urbanization and the COVID-19 pandemic.

COVID-19 and Urbanization

Urbanization is another leading global trend of the 21st century that substantially impacts social, psychological, and overall human health. Urban growth mainly takes place in developing cities. Approximately half of the population residing in large metropolitan cities suffers from a lack of housing, transport, poor sanitation, and exposure to high environmental pollution. These conditions make the urban zones epicenters of noncommunicable diseases [21]. The worldwide administration must guide policies to minimize rapid urbanization and urban development trends in order to protect and promote health.

The European Public Health Alliance (EPHA) warned that people living in metropolitan and polluted cities are at higher risk of SARS-CoV-2 infection [22]. According to the US Environmental Protection Agency (US-EPA), breathing air with a high concentration of NO_2 can negatively affect the human respiratory system [22]. Environmental pollutants reduce lung function and can cause coughs, bronchial asthma, wheezing, and lung inflammation. Subjects with prolonged exposure to air pollution and chronic lung and coronary artery diseases cannot fight against lung infections and have a high mortality rate. This is more likely seen in COVID-19 cases [23] in large metropolitan cities and urban areas.

SARS-CoV-2 infection is widely diffused in many European countries, particularly in the United Kingdom, Spain, and Germany. The European Environment Agency (EEA) has recently highlighted that the air quality index (AQI) is reflecting the potential impact of air quality on human health [24]. The AQI is based on environmental pollutants, including PM10, PM2.5, O_3, SO_2, and NO_2. These pollutants were mainly found in the most polluted areas of Italy and Europe [25]. At the same time, the fatality rate in these Italian regions was higher. The pollution in these Italian regions could be one factor for the increasing mortality rate due to the coronavirus [26].

In the United States, a country-level, comprehensive study estimates the relationship between long-term exposure to PM2.5 and COVID-19 mortality. An increase in $1 \ g/m^3$ of PM2.5 exposure was associated with a 15% increase in the COVID-19 mortality rate [27]. This analysis provides a timely relationship between exposure to air pollution and COVID-19 deaths in the United States.

In several urbanized areas of the world, air pollution patterns are changing with weather conditions and climate scenarios, significantly affecting respiratory health. The climate allied factors such as humidity, temperature, cloud cover, visibility, air pressure, and wind speed increase mortality and morbidity [28-29]. There is strong evidence that environmental pollution and weather conditions affect the incidence and mortality rates associated with viral epidemics [30]. Meo et al. (2020) [31] reported that weather events and the COVID-19 pandemic impact various regional levels. The authors identified an increase in relative humidity and temperatures associated with decreased daily cases and deaths due to the COVID-19 pandemic in different African countries. In addition, to present linkage and lessons on urbanization and the COVID-19 pandemic, it is essential to discuss the facts and figures based on the currently available scientific literature on the global situation of environmental pollution and the COVID-19 pandemic.

Environmental Pollution and the COVID-19 Pandemic

Environmental pollution can affect the respiratory airways through inhalation and exacerbate the susceptibility to respiratory virus infections [13]. An environment with high toxic pollutants and particular climatic conditions may promote the long-term existence of the viral particles in the environment. The polluted environment contains dust, fumes, gases, and particulate matter (PM). Air pollutants can travel from region to region, enter into the respiratory system and negatively affect human health (Figure 3.1). It would also favor an indirect diffusion of SARS-CoV-2, in addition to the direct distribution to individuals [32, 33].

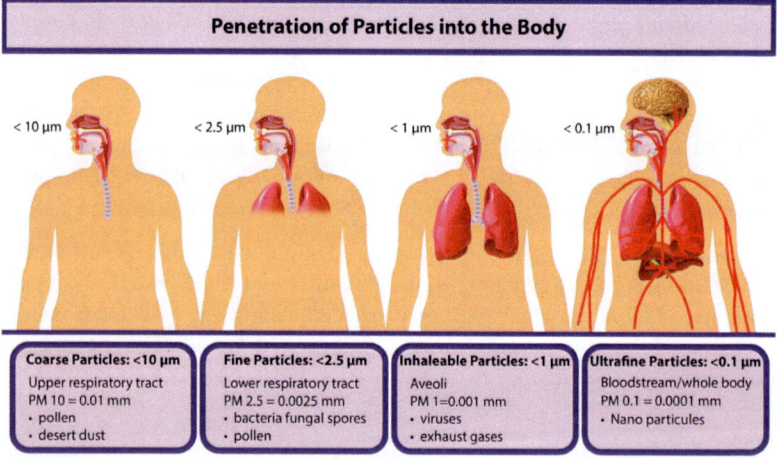

Figure 3.1. The penetration of particulate matter (PM) in the respiratory system.

Martelletti and Martelletti (2020) [34] have performed a study in the Northern regions of Italy, which were mainly affected by COVID-19 cases and deaths and had the highest concentrations of PM10 and PM2.5. The authors suggested that SARS-CoV-2 could find suitable transporters in air pollutant particles and become a cause of respiratory infections. Individuals residing in zones with high concentrations of air pollutants are more prone to developing respiratory diseases [35] and viral infections [36]. Environmental pollution impairs the first line of defense of the upper airways, mainly cilia, and causes respiratory illness [37].

Conticini et al. (2020) [38] reported that people living in large metropolitan cities are more prone to COVID-19 incidence and mortality due to their long-term exposure to pollution and deteriorated health status caused by air pollution. In China, Zhu et al. (2020) [39] investigated the relationship between environmental pollutants PM2.5, PM10, CO, NO_2, and O_3 and daily confirmed COVID-19 cases in about 120 cities. There was a significant positive association of the contaminants with COVID-19 confirmed cases. The study findings also support the hypothesis that environmental pollution can be an essential risk factor in the COVID-19 pandemic.

Ribeiro and Barros (2020) [40] conducted a study on environmental pollution and increased susceptibility to the COVID-19 pandemic. The findings revealed a positive association between PM10 and PM2.5 and SARS-CoV-2 cases. Chronic exposure to air pollutants impairs recovery and leads to more severe and lethal forms of the disease [38, 27].

Coccia (2020) [10, 11] investigated the mechanisms of transmission of COVID-19 in the environment. It was identified that the high transmission of COVID-19 in the specific climate was due to air pollution-to-human transmission and human-to-human transmission in the context of a high density of population. It was found that COVID-19 in North Italy has a high association with air pollution in cities having more than 100 days of air pollution exceeding the limits for PM10; however, cities having fewer than 100 days of air pollution showed a lower number of SARS-CoV-2 cases.

The SARS-CoV-2 infection continues to rise in various states of America, where 80% of the population live in urban areas that are also home to some of the enormous societal inequities in the world [41]. The chronic diseases associated with long-term exposure to air pollution appear to be allied with a higher vulnerability to severe COVID-19 outcomes [42, 43]. A recent study reported an increase in 1 $\mu g/m^3$ PM2.5 associated with an 8% increase in the COVID-19 death rate [27]. The literature also supports the hypothesis that short-term air pollution exposures interact with SARS-CoV-2 infections [44].

The science community has established a strong link between various environmental pollutants and an increasing number of SARS-CoV-2 cases and deaths. Setti et al. (2020a) [45] have analyzed the impact of airborne pollutants, including particulate matter (PM10), from the industrial areas. The findings show that SARS-CoV-2 can be attached to PM10 and can move from region to region. The evidence indicates that SARS-CoV-2 can be found on PM [45, 46]. The presence of SARS-CoV-2 on air pollutant PM10 might potentially be an early indicator of the COVID-19 pandemic [45-47]. Similar findings have also been reported by Conticini et al. (2020)

[38] in Italian regions with the highest levels of virus lethality in the world. Remarkably, both regions were amongst the most polluted areas of Europe; people living in high concentrations of air pollutants were more prone to developing chronic respiratory conditions. It was further summarized that a high level of environmental pollution was an additional co-factor of the SARS-CoV-2 lethality recorded in these areas.

Similarly, Frontera et al. (2020) [32] have established a relationship between environmental pollution PM2.5 and NO_2 with SARS-CoV-2 incidence and mortality. The potential mechanism is that chronic exposure to PM2.5 causes the overexpression of the alveolar angiotensin-converting enzyme 2 (ACE-2) receptor, which can increase the viral load in patients exposed to air pollutants. In turn, this would deplete ACE-2 receptors, impairing host defenses. Also, high NO_2 levels can cause severe SARS-CoV-2 in ACE-2 depleted lungs, with poor outcomes.

In contrast to these findings, Bontempi (2020) [48] has reported that direct correlations between high levels of particulate matter and the diffusion of SARS-CoV-2 are not evident. In another study, Bontempi et al. (2020) [49, 50] concluded that the current pandemic's diffusion patterns are caused by a multiplicity of environmental, economic, and social factors and not simply due to environmental pollution.

Bashir et al. (2020) [51] investigated the association of PM2.5, PM10, SO_2, NO_2, Pb, VOCs, and CO, with COVID-19 cases in California. It was found that PM10, PM2.5, SO_2, NO_2, and CO levels showed a significant correlation with the COVID-19 pandemic. On the other hand, Wu et al. 2020 [27] assessed whether long-term average exposure to PM2.5 in the USA was associated with an increased risk of COVID-19 deaths. COVID-19 death counts were collected for more than 3,000 counties, with about 98% of the population across the country. Furthermore, Liang et al. (2020) [52] conducted a nationwide cross-sectional study and determined the association between long-term county-level exposure to PM2.5, NO_2, and O_3 and COVID-19 case-fatality and mortality rates. The authors included 3,122 counties and analyzed the outcome. The authors found positive associations between long-term exposure to NO_2 and the COVID-19 case-fatality and mortality rates.

In England, Travaglio et al. (2020) [53] reported that poor air quality due to nitrogen oxide and sulfur dioxide was associated with an increased number of COVID-19-related deaths across England. Also, Li et al. (2020) [54] investigated the effect of air pollutants, including PM2.5, PM10, NO_2, and CO, and meteorological variables such as temperature, temperature difference, and sunshine duration on the COVID-19 incidence. It was noticed that AQI, PM2.5, NO_2, and temperature could promote the coronavirus.

Zhu et al. (2020) [39] assessed the relationship between ambient air pollutants, PM2.5, PM10, SO_2, CO, NO_2, and O_3, with confirmed cases of SARS-CoV-2 in over 100 cities. It was found that a 10-µg/m³ increase in PM2.5, PM10, NO_2, and O_3 was related to a 2.24, 1.76%, 6.94%, and 4.76% increase in the daily SARS-CoV-2 confirmed cases, respectively.

On the other hand, Ogen (2020) [44] has investigated the effect of long-term exposure to NO_2 on COVID-19 fatality. The author recorded the data from 66 regions of France, Germany, Italy, and Spain. It was concluded that chronic exposure to NO_2 could be an essential contributor to the high COVID-19 fatality rates observed in these regions. However, this conclusion was questioned by Chudnovsky (2020) [55], who stated that only two months of exposure to NO_2 could not be considered as a long-term exposure. Chudnovsky (2020) [55] further noted that there were low fatality rates in countries like Taiwan with much higher air concentrations of NO_2. The response of Ogen (2020) [44] was that his results simply showed that the highest number of cases were observed in highly polluted areas of Europe.

Bilal et al. (2020) [56] suggested that PM10, NO_2, O_3, and CO emissions are the main determinants of the COVID-19 pandemic in the South American region. The authors further reported that environmental pollutants could cause numerous chronic illnesses and are detrimental to the human immune system. Ecological contaminants significantly contributed to the spread of COVID-19 in the region. Wu et al. (2020) [27] empirically analyzed data from more than 300 USA counties indicated that long-term exposure to fine particulate matter increases the chances of deaths by up to 15% and is responsible for a 20 times higher death rate from viral illnesses such as COVID-19. Bilal et al. (2021) [56] and Xu et al. (2020) [57] also supported similar findings by pointing out that PM2.5 and PM10 are vital contributors to the spread of COVID-19 in high pollutant countries. It was identified that environmental pollution is a leading contributing factor for the COVID-19 pandemic.

In a few US states, there has been an increased number of wildfire incidences in 2020. The literature also establishes some links and connections, regarding this, to the COVID-19 pandemic.

Wildfire Allied Pollution and the COVID-19 Pandemic

Wildfire occurrences have a drastic impact on the weather conditions and environment and develop a hazardous situation for human health and living organisms. Wildfire allied environmental pollution is highly toxic. It can cause significant wide-ranging damage to the regional environment and weather conditions while also facilitating the transmission of microorganisms and diseases. The wildfire air contains smoke, gases, dust, fine particles, and particulate matter due to the burning of plants, wood, buildings, and other materials. Wildfire smoke is a mixture of "carbon dioxide, carbon monoxide, nitrogen oxides," particulate matter, hydrocarbons, and other organic compounds [58]. The pollutants travel from the actual site of the wildfire over the country, causing various health problems.

Wildfire allied pollution poses various human health hazards and economic challenges. There is a relationship between wildfire smoke and particulate matter (PM2.5) exposures with various respiratory diseases, cardiovascular illnesses and mortality. The respiratory morbidity includes "bronchial asthma, chronic obstructive pulmonary disease, bronchitis, and pneumonia." Those in the population susceptible to wildfire smoke exposure include middle-aged and older adults with acute or chronic respiratory and cardiovascular diseases, along with pregnant women and fetuses [59]. The same group of people are also susceptible to SARS-COV-2 infection [60, 61].

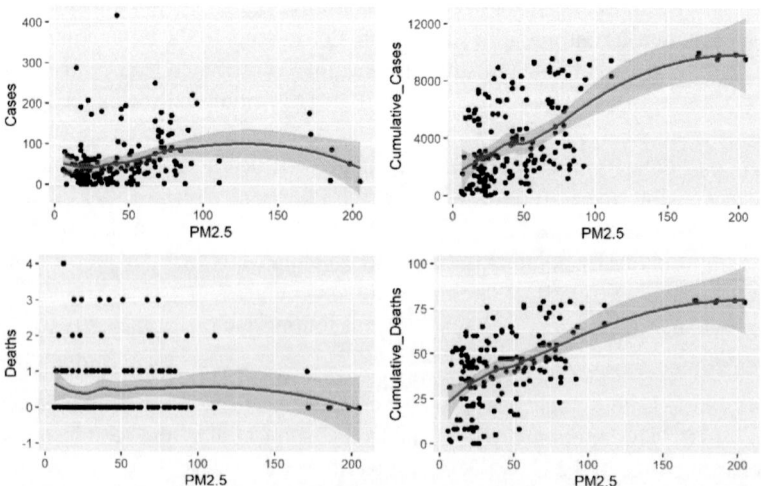

Figure 3.2: Relationship of PM2.5 with cases, deaths, cumulative cases, and deaths.

[Adopted after permission obtained from the author and publisher] [62].

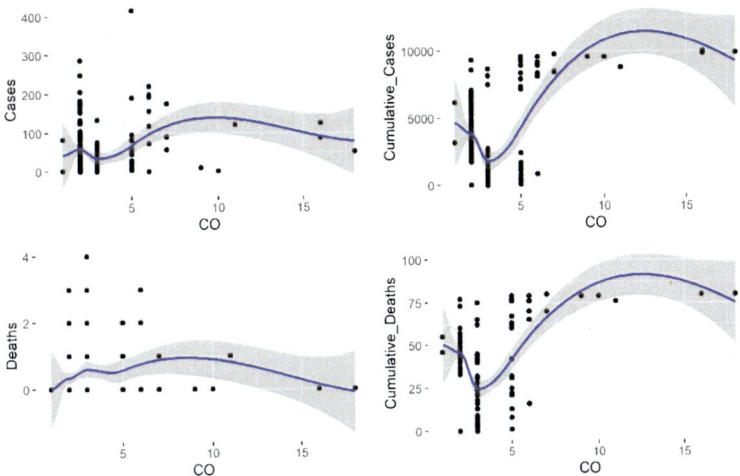

Figure 3.3: Relationship of CO with cases, deaths, cumulative cases, and deaths. [Adopted after permission obtained from the author and publisher] [62].

The rising incidences of wildfires in the surrounding areas of San Francisco, California caused pollution, which posed a significant threat to social and environmental development, the health care system, and economies. The primary pollutant components of a wildfire are smoke, particulate matter (PM2.5), and carbon monoxide (CO). Meo et al. (2020) [62] study showed the increasing epidemiological trends of COVID-19 cases and deaths with wildfire allied environmental pollutants PM2.5 and carbon monoxide in San Francisco, California.

Literature has acknowledged that wildfire allied environmental pollution increases the incidence and mortality of SARS-COV-2 infection. Kan et al. (2005) [63] reported that the coronavirus outbreak increased by a prominent 6% with a relative risk of mortality for every ten micrograms per cubic meter increase in the mean of total respirable particulate matter (PM10), which also comprises PM2.5 and larger particles. Similarly, Croft et al. (2018) [64] demonstrated an increased hospitalization rate for culture-negative pneumonia and influenza linked with increased PM2.5 concentrations among residents of metropolitan urban areas of New York, USA. In another study, Croft et al. (2020) [65] reported that short-term increases in particulate matter (PM2.5) from traffic and various combustion sources are a potential risk for increased rates of influenza hospitalizations and hospital visits. The authors further established that biomass burning was associated with laboratory-confirmed cases of influenza.

Meo et al. [62] conducted a study, investigating the association between wildfire allied pollutants, PM2.5, CO, and ozone with daily cases and deaths due to SARS-CoV 2 infection in 10 counties in California which were affected by wildfire. After the wildfire, PM2.5, O_3, and CO concentrations were increased, and the number of cases and deaths due to COVID-19 markedly increased. The results revealed a significant positive correlation between the wildfire allied environmental pollutants and SARS-CoV-2 daily cases, cumulative cases, and deaths. SARS-CoV-2 can be easily transported through air and air pollutants. Air is a highly suitable transmission method through which microbial agents may move around the environment and various regions; bacteria, fungi, viruses, parasites, and spores can be bioaerosol components. The particulate environmental matters play a role as carriers of numerous microorganisms, including viruses. The particulate matters increase the effectiveness of the virus spread and provide a suitable environment for its persistence.

Moreover, PM2.5 and microorganisms can be easily inhaled deep into the lungs, mainly smaller than 2.5 microns (PM2.5 and ultrafine particulate matter). This facilitates the virus to enter into the respiratory tract and cause infections. The discussion is supported by some evidence that exposure to PM pollution is exceptionally high in wildfire regions, where an excess of COVID-19 cases and deaths have been reported. PM exposure has been causally linked to several organ dysfunctions, mostly involving the respiratory system and the severe course of COVID-19.

The literature has established some pathophysiological and epidemiological links between PM exposure and viral infections. Moreover, there is an association between airborne pollution and COVID-19 incidences. Environmental pollution particulate matters act as a carrier of the infection, impair immunity, make people more susceptible to pathogens, and worsen the disease's pathogenic factor. These are the few pieces of evidence that strengthen the linkage between the wildfire pollutants' particulate matter PM2.5 and carbon monoxide (CO) on the epidemiological dynamics of COVID-19 cases and mortality. The study findings indicate that particulate matter (PM2.5) is the best carrier or transport vector for the SARS-COV-2 virus. Moreover, carbon monoxide is a highly toxic gas that can damage the lungs. This mechanism supports the hypothesis that the wildfire pollutants' particulate matter (PM2.5) and carbon monoxide resulted in increased SARS-COV-2 cases and deaths in the wildfire regions.

Conclusions

Environmental pollution has a significant impact on human health. Environmental pollutants are the main determinants of the COVID-19 pandemic in various regions of the world. The numerous studies and findings confirm that higher environmental pollution has contributed significantly to the spread of COVID-19. The increased exposure to environmental pollutants causes a significant risk of getting infected, especially amongst older adults. The metropolitan cities with higher environmental pollution have higher infection levels and deaths due to exceedingly high particulate matter or ozone levels. The literature strongly suggests that environmental pollution is one of the determining factors increasing the spread of COVID-19.

Moreover, the geographical, demographic, environmental, and weather conditions influence infectious diseases, especially in large metropolitan cities and urban areas. Thus, substantial evidence supports a clear association between concentrations of various environmental pollutants and human respiratory viruses interacting to adversely affect the respiratory system. The findings have outcomes for policymakers and health officials about the impact of environmental pollution on the epidemiological and pathological trends of new daily cases and deaths due to the COVID-19 pandemic. The meteorological and health officials must implement and adapt policies to minimize environmental pollution and enhance awareness in planning to fight against environmental and pandemic situations, both at regional and international levels.

References

1. Meo SA, Azeem MA, Ghori MG, Subhan MM. Lung function and surface electromyography of intercostal muscles in cement mill workers. Int J Occup Med Environ Health. 2002;15 (3): 279-87.

2. Prabhat K Rai. Particulate Matter and Its Size Fractionation, Biomagnetic Monitoring of Particulate Matter, 2016; 1-13.

3. World Health Organization. Air pollution Available at http://origin. who.int/airpollution/en/Cited date Feb 12, 2020.

4. Manisalidis I, Stavropoulou E, Stavropoulos A, Bezirtzoglou E. Environmental and health impacts of air pollution: a review. Front Public Health. 2020;8:14. doi:10.3389/fpubh.2020.00014.

5. Eissenberg T., Kanj S.S., Shihadeh AL Treat COVID-19 as though it is airborne: it may Be. AANA J. (Am. Assoc. Nurse Anesth.) 2020;88:29-30.

6. Pereira IG, Guerin JM, Junior AGS, Distante C, Garcia GS, Goncalves LM. Forecasting Covid-19 dynamics in Brazil: a data-driven approach. arXiv. 2020; 2005: 09475.

7. Huang C, Wang Y, Li X, et al. Clinical features of patients infected with 2019 novel coronavirus in Wuhan, China. Lancet. 2020; 395 (10223): 497-506.

8. Haque SE, Rahman M. Association between temperature, humidity, and COVID-19 outbreaks in Bangladesh. Environ Sci Pol. 2020; 114: 253-255. doi:10.1016/j.envsci.2020.08.012.

9. Bashir MF, Ma B, Komal B, Bashir MA, Tan D. Correlation between climate indicators and COVID-19 pandemic in New York, USA. Sci Total Environ. 2020;728:138835. doi:10.1016/j.scitotenv.2020.138835.

10. Coccia M. An index to quantify the environmental risk of exposure to future epidemics of the COVID-19 and similar viral agents: theory and practice. Environ Res. 2020; 191:110155. doi:10.1016/j.envres. 2020.110155.

11. Coccia M. Factors determining the diffusion of COVID-19 and suggested strategy to prevent future accelerated viral infectivity similar to COVID. Sci Total Environ. 2020;138474. doi:10.1016/j.scitotenv. 2020.138474.

12. Morawska L., Cao J. Airborne transmission of SARS-CoV-2: the world should face reality. Environ. Int. 2020;139:105730.

13. Ciencewicki J., Jaspers I. Air pollution and respiratory viral infection. Inhal. Toxicol. 2007;19:1135–1146.

14. Pothirat C., Chaiwong W., Liwsrisakun C., Bumroongkit C., Deesomchok A., Theerakittikul T., Limsukon A., Tajarernmuang P., Phetsuk N. Acute effects of air pollutants on daily mortality and hospitalizations due to cardiovascular and respiratory diseases. J. Thorac. Dis. 2019;11:3070–3083.

15. Su W., Wu X., Geng X., Zhao X., Liu Q., Liu T. The short-term effects of air pollutants on influenza-like illness in Jinan, China. BMC Publ. Health. 2019; 19: 1319.

16. Chen C.W.S., Hsieh Y.H., Su H.C., Wu J.J. Causality test of fine ambient particles and human Influenza in Taiwan: age group-specific disparity and geographic heterogeneity. Environ. Int. 2018;111:354–361.

17. Chen G., Zhang W., Li S., Zhang Y., Williams G., Huxley R., Ren H., Cao W., Guo Y. The impact of fine ambient particles on influenza transmission and the modification effects of temperature in China: a multi-city study. Environ. Int. 2017;98:82–88.

18. Ye Q., Fu J.F., Mao J.H., Shang S.Q. Haze is a risk factor contributing to the rapid spread of the respiratory syncytial virus in children. Environ. Sci. Pollut. Res. Int. 2016; 23: 20178-20185.

19. Nenna R., Evangelisti M., Frassanito A., Scagnolari C., Pierangeli A., Antonelli G., Nicolai A., Arima S., Moretti C., Papoff P., Villa M.P., Midulla F. Respiratory syncytial virus bronchiolitis, weather conditions and air pollution in an Italian urban area: an observational study. Environ. Res. 2017;158:188–193.

20. Zhao Q., Chen H., Yang T., Rui W., Liu F., Zhang F., Zhao Y., Ding W. Direct effects of airborne PM2.5 exposure on macrophage polarization. Biochim. Biophys. Acta. 2016;1860: 2835-2843.

21. World Health Organization. Urban Health. https://www.who.int/health-topics/urban-health. Cited date Jan 2, 2021.

22. European Public Health Alliance. Clean air – latest developments COVID–19; [cited Mar 16, 2020]. Available from: Epha.org/coronavirus-threat-greater--for-polluted-cities/

23. Lerner S. Million people in the US could die if coronavirus goes unchecked; [cited Mar 17, 2020]. Available from: https://theintercept.com/2020/03/17/coronavirus-air-pollution/.

24. Barbrioglio E. Europe's 100 most polluted cities; [cited Feb 29, 2020]. Available from: https://www.forbes.com/sites/emanuelabarbiroglio/2020/02/29/cities-in-polandanditaly-among-europes-100-mostpolluted/#77eaacd058fd.

25. Qin C, Zhou L, Hu Z, Zhang S, Yang S, Tao Y, et al. Dysregulation of immune response in patients with COVID19 in Wuhan, China. Clin Infect Dis 2020;71(15):762-768 doi.org/10.1093/cid/ciaa248.

26. Godin M. Why is Italy's Coronavirus outbreak so bad?; [cited Mar 10, 2020]. Available from: https://time.com/5799586/italy-coronavirus-outbreak/.

27. Wu X, Nethery RC, Sabbath BM, Braun D, Dominici F. Exposure to air pollution and COVID-19 mortality in the United States: A nationwide cross-sectional study. medRxiv. 2020:2020.04.05.20054502; 10.1101/2020.04.05.20054502.

28. Abe T, Tokuda Y, Ohde S, Ishimatsu S, Nakamura T, Birrer RB. The relationship of short-term air pollution and weather to ED visits for asthma in Japan. Am J Emerg Med 2009; 27: 153-159.

29. Ikaheimo TM, Juvonen R, Jokelainen J, Harju T, Peitso A, Bloigu A, et al. Cold temperature and low humidity are associated with increased

occurrence of respiratory tract infections. Respir Med 2009;103: 456-462.

30. Analitis A, Di Donato F, Scortichini M, Lanki T, Basagana X, Ballester F. synergistic effects of ambient temperature and air pollution on health in Europe: results from the PHASE project. Int J Environ Res Public Health 2018;15(9):1856.

31. Meo SA, Abukhalaf AA, Alomar AA, Aljudi TW, Bajri HM, Sami W, Akram J, Akram SJ, Hajjar W. Impact of weather conditions on incidence and mortality of COVID-19 pandemic in Africa. Eur Rev Med Pharmacol Sci. 2020 Sep;24(18):9753-9759. doi: 10.26355/ eurrev_202009_23069. PMID: 33015822.

32. Frontera A., Martin C., Vlachos K., Sgubin G. Regional air pollution persistence links to COVID-19 infection zoning. J. Infect. 2020; S0163–4453(20):30173–30180.

33. Frontera A., Cianfanelli L., Vlachos K., Landoni G., Cremona G. Severe air pollution links to higher mortality in COVID-19 patients: the "double-hit" hypothesis. J. Infect. 2020; S0163–4453(20):30285–30291.

34. Martelletti L., Martelletti P. Air pollution and the novel covid-19 disease: a putative disease risk factor. SN compr. Clin. Med. Apr. 2020;15:1–5.

35. Marquès M., Domingo J.L., Nadal M., Schuhmacher M. Health risks for the population living near petrochemical industrial complexes. 2. Adverse effects other than cancer. Sci. Total Environ. 2020 (in press)

36. Xie J., Teng J., Fan Y., Xie R., Shen A. The short-term effects of air pollutants on hospitalizations for respiratory disease in Hefei, China. Int. J. Biometeorol. 2019;63:315–326.

37. Cao Y., Chen M., Dong D., Xie S., Liu M. Environmental pollutants damage airway epithelial cell cilia: implications for the prevention of obstructive lung diseases. Thorac. Cancer. 2020;11:505–510.

38. Conticini E., Frediani B., Caro D. Can atmospheric pollution be considered a co-factor in an extremely high level of SARS-CoV-2 lethality in Northern Italy? Environ. Pollut. 2020;261:114465.

39. Zhu Y., Xie J., Huang F., Cao L. Association between short-term exposure to air pollution and COVID-19 infection: evidence from China. Sci. Total Environ. 2020;727.

40. Ribeiro A.I., Barros H. 2020. Association between COVID-19 Infections and Air Pollution: Evidence from Portugal. (unpublished data).

41. Josiah L. Kephart, Ione Avila-Palencia, Usama Bilal, Nelson Gouveia, Waleska T. Caiaffa, and Ana V. Diez Roux. COVID-19, Ambient Air Pollution, and Environmental Health Inequities in Latin American Cities. J Urban Health. 2021: 1-5. doi: 10.1007/s11524-020-00509-8.

42. CDC COVID-19 Response Team. Preliminary estimates of the prevalence of selected underlying health conditions among patients with coronavirus disease 2019 — United States, February 12–March 28, 2020.; 2020. 10.15585/mmwr.mm6913e2.

43. Onder G, Rezza G, Case-Fatality Rate BS. Characteristics of patients dying to COVID-19 in Italy. JAMA - J Am Med Assoc. March 2020; 10.1001/jama.2020.4683.

44. Ogen Y. Assessing nitrogen dioxide (NO_2) levels as a contributing factor to coronavirus (COVID-19) fatality. Sci Total Environ. 2020;726:138605. doi:10.1016/j.scitotenv.2020.138605.

45. Setti L, Passarini F, de-Gennaro G, Di Gilio A, Palmisano J, Buono P, Fornari G, Perrone MG, Piazzalunga A, Barbieri P. Evaluation of the Potential Relationship between Particulate Matter (PM) Pollution and COVID-19 Infection Spread in Italy. BMJ Open. Available at:

46. Setti L., Passarini F., De Gennaro G., Barbieri P., Pallavicini A., Ruscio M., Piscitelli P., Colao A., Miani A. Searching for SARS-COV-2 on particulate matter: a possible early indicator of COVID-19 epidemic recurrence. Int. J. Environ. Res. Publ. Health. 2020;17:E2986.

47. Setti L., Passarini F., De Gennaro G., Barbieri P., Perrone M.G., Borelli M., Palmisani J., Di Gilio A., Piscitelli P., Miani A. Airborne transmission route of COVID-19: why 2 meters/6 feet of inter-personal distance could not Be enough. Int. J. Environ. Res. Publ. Health. 2020;17:2932.

48. Bontempi E. First data analysis about possible COVID-19 virus airborne diffusion due to air particulate matter (PM): the case of Lombardy (Italy) Environ. Res. 2020;186:109639.

49. Bontempi E. Commercial exchanges instead of air pollution as a possible origin of COVID-19 initial diffusion phase in Italy: more efforts are necessary to address interdisciplinary research. Environ. Res. 2020 (in press)

50. Bontempi E., Vergalli S., Squazzoni F. Understanding COVID-19 diffusion requires an interdisciplinary, multi-dimensional approach. Environ. Res. 2020.

51. Bashir MF, Ma B, Shahbaz M, Jiao Z. The nexus between environmental tax and carbon emissions with the roles of environmental technology

and financial development. PLoS One. 2020;15(11):e0242412. doi:10.1371/journal.pone.0242412.

52. Liang D., Shi L., Zhao J., Liu P., Schwartz J., Gao S., Sarnat J., Liu Y., Ebelt S., Scovronick N., Chang H.H. medRxiv; 2020 May 7. Urban Air Pollution May Enhance COVID-19 Case-Fatality and Mortality Rates in the United States. 2020.05.04.20090746.

53. Travaglio M., Yu Y., Popovic R., Santos Leal N., Martins L.M. MedRxiv; 2020. Links between Air Pollution and COVID-19 in England.

54. Li H., Xu X.L., Dai D.W., Huang Z.Y., Ma Z., Guan Y.J. Air Pollution and temperature are associated with increased COVID-19 incidence: a time-series study. Int. J. Infect. Dis. 2020; S1201–9712.

55. Chudnovsky A.A. Letter to the editor regarding Ogen Y 2020 paper: "Assessing nitrogen dioxide (NO_2) levels as a contributing factor to coronavirus (COVID-19) fatality. Sci. Total Environ. 2020;6:139236.

56. Bilal, Bashir MF, Komal B, Benghoul M, Bashir MA, Tan D. Nexus Between the COVID-19 Dynamics and Environmental Pollution Indicators in South America. Risk Manag Healthc Policy. 2021 Jan 8;14:67-74.

57. Xu H., Yan C., Fu Q., Xiao K., Yu Y., Han D., Wang W., Cheng J. Possible environmental effects on the spread of COVID-19 in China. Sci. Total Environ. 2020;731:139211.

58. Urbanski SP, Hao WM, Baker S. Chemical Composition of Wildland Fire Smoke, in Arbaugh M, Riebau A, Andersen C (Eds.), Developments in Environmental Science, Elsevier BV. 2009; 79-107.

59. Cascio WE. Wildland fire smoke and human health. Sci Total Environ, 2018; 624: 586-595.

60. Madjid M, Safavi-Naeini P, Solomon SD, Vardeny O. Potential Effects of Coronaviruses on the Cardiovascular System: A Review. JAMA Cardiol 2020; 5: 831-840.

61. Meo SA, Alhowikan AM, Al-Khlaiwi T, Meo IM, Halepoto DM, Iqbal M, Usmani AM, Hajjar W, Ahmed N. Novel coronavirus 2019-nCoV: prevalence, biological and clinical characteristics comparison with SARS-CoV and MERS-CoV. Eur Rev Med Pharmacol Sci 2020; 24: 2012-2019.

62. Meo SA, Abukhalaf AA, Alomar AA, Alessa OM, Sami W, Klonoff DC. Effect of environmental pollutants PM-2.5, carbon monoxide, and ozone on the incidence and mortality of SARS-COV-2 infection in

ten wildfire-affected counties in California. Sci Total Environ. 2021 ; 757:143948. doi: 10.1016/j.scitotenv.

63. Kan HD, Chen BH, Fu CW, Yu SZ, Mu LN. Relationship between ambient air pollution and daily mortality of SARS in Beijing. Biomed Environ Sci. 2005; 18:1-4.

64. Croft DP, Zhang W, Lin S, Thurston SW, Hopke PK, Masiol M, Thevenet-Morrison K, Van Wijngaarden E, Utell M, Rich D. The association between respiratory infection and air pollution in the setting of air quality policy and economic change. Ann Am Thorac. Soc 2018; 16: 321-330.

65. Croft DP, Zhang W, Lin S, Thurston SW, Hopke PK, van Wijngaarden E, Squizzato S, Masiol M, Utell MJ, Rich DQ. Associations between Source-Specific Particulate Matter and Respiratory Infections in New York State Adults. Environ Sci Technol. 2020; 54: 975-984.

Climate Change and Covid-19: Linkages and Lessons

Khalid Mahmood Shafi | Ruhaab Khalid

Summary

Climate change is a leading global health hazard of the 21st century. Due to the complex combination and effects of biological, chemical, and physical processes, the extent to which the changing climate may influence health remains unknown and under-researched. The world is now facing the prime crisis of the COVID-19 pandemic. The decisions taken by individuals and governments will shape the world in the coming decades. They will change our health care systems and societies, economies, politics, and culture. It is time to realize how to overcome the instant threat. It also needs to be determined whether the world will accept the living environment once the pandemic passes. Climate change may suffer in the post-pandemic period due to multiple reasons, including economic priorities and national/international donors' policy priorities regarding climate change-related funds. The viability and preferential treatment of climate change organizations must remain intact, adopting international laws and conventions regarding climate change. World leaders and organizations have a shared responsibility for developing and maintaining solid global competency to check communicable diseases and climate change. This competency comprises guaranteeing the availability of funds to fill the gaps in epidemic preparedness and climate change control. These measures will protect humanity and lead to a safer and more secure world. Timely climate change policies should be promoted to control the spread of infectious diseases, such as the COVID-19 pandemic.

Keywords: Climate Change, Covid-19, Human Health, Linkages, and Lessons

Introduction

These unprecedented times during the COVID-19 pandemic, comprising bewilderment at all tiers of policy formulation and assorted stages of lockdowns, have given the world the much-needed energy and time for introspection. Although the situation worsened with numerous cases and deaths during the pandemic, there are also indications about how human inactivity positively affected Mother Earth. Seeing wildlife regain space, a clearer atmosphere, and reduced pollution in waters seemed to be a reenergizing situation for the blighted Mother Nature. This pandemic has unveiled the interrelationship between nature and human health. Protecting the planet and the climate is crucial to prevent another pathogen crippling civilization. To care for humanity, it is essential to care about the climate. The science literature demonstrates that about 60% of human infectious diseases such as bird flu, swine flu, and mad cow disease originated from animals [1]. It is strongly believed that there is an acute need to eliminate the illegal wildlife trade, curtail deforestation and restrict ecosystem destruction as it enhances the risk of environmental pollution and transmitting various diseases from wildlife to humans. The COVID-19 pandemic has established beyond a shadow of a doubt that nature and humans share the same destiny and are much more linked than anyone could have imagined earlier.

After flattening the COVID trajectory curve, it will be more important to reconsider the global climate change policies adopted by the major nations against the backdrop of pandemic policies. All three major contributors of planet-warming gases have a different trajectory. The European Union (EU) has laid down a vision of a green future. It has a package worth 800$ billion that would facilitate the transition from fossil fuels and ensure energy efficiency. The Green Deal is viewed as a political cudgel against political opponents. In the USA, the divide between Republicans and Democrats is quite visible. Environmental laws are being relaxed in the COVID-19 environment, and data are not adequately quoted. However, the international community has pledged to re-join the Paris Agreement and vow that the United States would "take a back seat to no one when it comes to fighting climate change"[2]. China has given the green light to build new coal plants. However, it declined to set ambitious economic targets, which is a relief for environmentalists as it does not eliminate, but lessens, the pressures to speed up quick industrialization. The need of the hour is to have a uniform collective non-myopic approach in dealing with dual international pressing agendas.

The COVID-19 pandemic was considered a short-term relief that gave breathing space to the planet; however, on the other hand, a counterproductive effect on international climate legislation and cooperation is also visible. World leaders agreed to reduce emissions to net-zero but disagreed on the transition speed. Against the backdrop of COVID-19, it is now vital for nations to use this opportunity of economic recovery for plans that are climate efficient and not reliant on the erstwhile fossil fuel companies. The climate crisis, coupled with this pandemic, has now amply demonstrated the trend in which societies are based; unsustainable on a planet with finite resources since we do not have the luxury of another planet. "Pathogens are inevitable, but that they turn into pandemics is not," similarly "Climate change is inevitable, but how we shape it is not" [3].

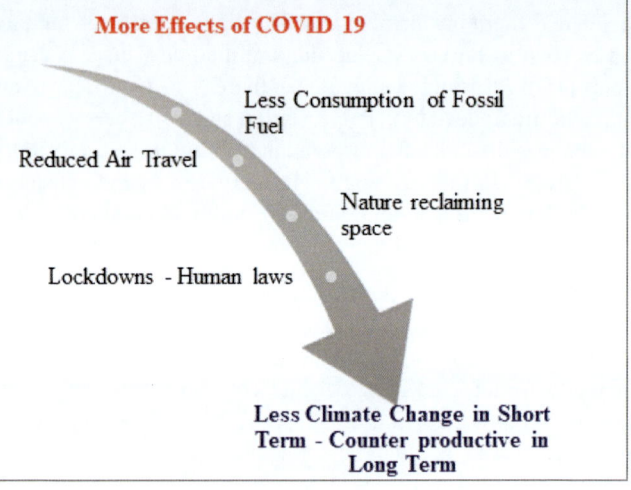

Figure 4.1: COVID-19 Pandemic and Climate Change.

The severe acute respiratory syndrome coronavirus (SARS-CoV-2) infection did not have appropriate medical treatment, and vaccination production has just been started. Preventive strategies were adopted in closing industries, limiting transportations, home restrictions, social distancing, and varied concepts of lockdowns adopted by different nations as per their environments. Despite having an immediate positive impact on the air quality, less emission of greenhouse gases, repair of the ozone layer, and less fuel demand, in the intermediate timeframe, adverse effects were visible in the form of violation of climate laws, diversion of funds from the climate crisis to address health issues, fewer demonstrations by climate activists, etc. It is generally perceived that although immediately after the COVID-19 pandemic, less climate change was observed, subsequently, in the long term, it will prove to be counterproductive as the world returns to normal without considering the lessons (Figure 4.1). Instead of a global approach to a phenomenon that knows no boundaries, nations will adopt their systems with additional focus on health care in the short term, rather than climate concerns in the long term.

The academicians and scholars do agree that before this lethal pandemic, there was already a pandemic, i.e., climate change, which in one way or another is still more lethal for human life. The climate crisis and the COVID-19 pandemic are pressing emergencies faced by the world, but the former is different, due to its severe and slow nature [4]. Furthermore, the COVID-19 pandemic could potentially be controlled with vaccines. However, if Antarctica melts, deforestation occurs in Alaska and Canada, and the lungs of the world – the Amazon forests – turn from Carbon sink to sources, then there is no going back. Between 2030-2050, climate change is predicted to cause about 250,000 additional deaths per annum from undernourishment, malarial parasites, diarrhea, and increased temperature stress [5]. The estimated loss to health is between two to four billion US Dollars. Human health in specific and the planet, in general, would suffer indubitably due to variations in the global environment, such as ozone layer depletion, environmental pollution, and unplanned urbanization and industrialization. This could also become a catalyst in the eruption of a second and third wave of pandemics. This combination could be more lethal than the combined nuclear arsenals of the world.

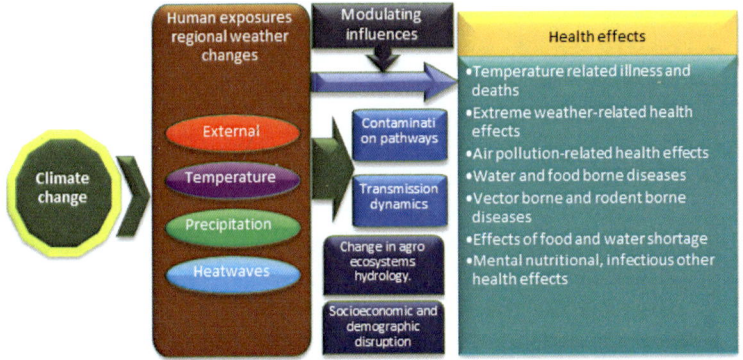

Fig 4.2: Mechanism of climate change.

The rise in climate change originates from industrial development. The enormous release of carbon dioxide, carbon monoxide, and other toxic gases during the industrial revolution, which resulted in greenhouse effects, surrounds the entire world and has developed health hazards [6]. Increasing worldwide temperatures, and the growing occurrences of extreme climatic events, result in fluctuations in the seasonality, geography, and intensity of infectious diseases [7, 8]. The mechanism by which climate changes affect human health and human life is summarized in Figure 4.2.

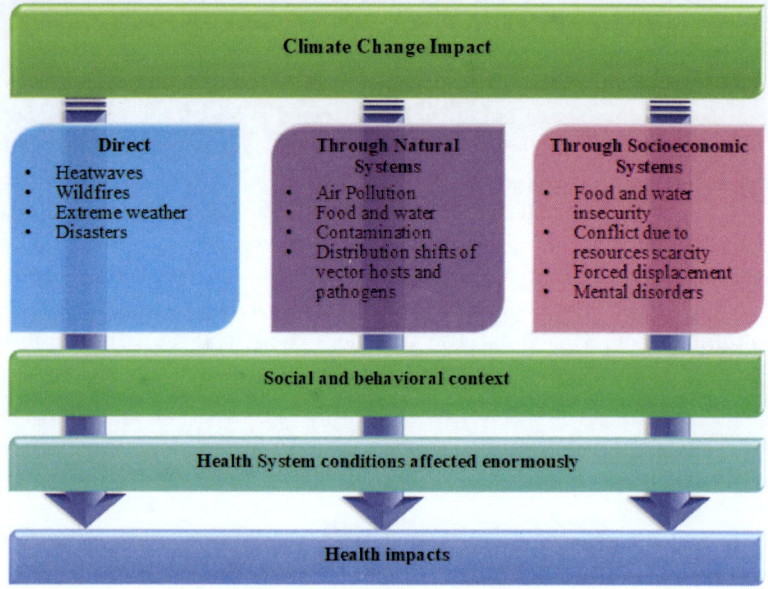

Fig 4.3: Mechanism by which climate change affects human health.

The sudden appearance of the COVID-19 pandemic has caused havoc worldwide, but it has also amplified the environmental aspects. Unlike climatic change, its lethality and impact are sudden. Before COVID-19, the human race has suffered from many pandemics in recent times, e.g., influenza (Swine Flu) in 2009, poliomyelitis in 2014, Ebola (West Africa in 2014), Zika Virus (2016), and Ebola (2019) in the Congo. The COVID-19 pandemic is considered the sixth major viral outbreak. The World Health Organization declared it a Public Health Emergency of International Concern (PHEIC) on January 30, 2020. The linkage between climate and its effect on human health is discussed below [9].

The COVID-19 Pandemic and Climate Change

The COVID-19 pandemic has affected climate change; whether it is positive or negative is debatable and will be revealed with time and adopted actions. "The pandemic that cleared skies, and halted cities, is not slowing global warming" [9]. However, pre-COVID-19, the thought of shutting down smoke factories, a sudden fall in emissions, and restricting billions of people to their homes was unthinkable.

The greatest challenge to humanity in the Post-World War II era was the war on terror in the aftermath of 9/11. However, COVID-19 has surpassed the war on terror. The COVID-19 pandemic is regarded as posing the biggest challenge to human beings and critical international health disasters. The COVID-19 pandemic is globally devastating, making world economies decelerate due to stringent lockdown measures. Nevertheless, the pandemic has some bearing upon the environment in a riveting way, too. As the COVID-19 infection unfurled worldwide, borders became meaningless, as it is for climate change. COVID-19 is affecting the lives of millions of people and the environment also. Lockdowns and social distancing brought the pollution-emitting industries and transport to almost a halt, reducing carbon dioxide gas and human mobility, improving air quality, and diverting wild faunae to visit the cities.

The environmental effects of lockdown movement restrictions have been beneficial so far. Production of wastage from industries has decreased phenomenally due to the closure of industries. The usage of fossil fuels and other energy sources has been reduced due to the minimum demand. This resulted in the recovery of natural ecosystems [11]. The use of hydrocarbons and, subsequently, energy demand, has dramatically reduced by almost 85% due to economic slowdown and closure of industries. The shrink in oil demand has worsened market imbalances and led to crude oil prices touching the rearmost level in over two decades. The decrease in electricity demand due to lockdown and the overall change in global energy is enormous [12].

It is expected that greenhouse gas emissions may fall by more than 8% or 2.6 Gt Carbon Dioxide in 2020) [13] than recorded in any previous years. COVID-19 related restrictions, imposed by governments worldwide since March 2020, drove a decline of daily global greenhouse emissions by as much as 17% by early April [14]. The percentage of greenhouse gas is expected to decline as the years 2020-21 progress. The trend may not continue in future years as the world returns to normalcy. However, the world has to act to bring greenhouse gas to net zero levels by 2050.

The question arises: after this global recession, what will happen? Greenhouse gas emissions are expected to increase rapidly where climate promoters will come to face the real problems. GHG emissions have increased considerably over the past decades; only the year 2020 saw decrease, and then a significant and unmatched surge is anticipated from 2021 onwards [14].

Climate change has a profound effect on air pollution, and air pollution is an alarming health danger. Every year, air pollution kills approximately 7 million people and is considered to be responsible for 1/3 of all mortalities, from thrombosis to lung carcinoma [15], and cardiac disease [16]. More than 90% of the global population live in places where the World Health Organization (WHO) outdoor air quality guideline levels are unmet [15, 17]. It has been reported that in the last few years, about five hundred tons of carbon dioxide gas have been generated. In 2019, forty billion tons of carbon dioxide was produced per $88 billion of the global GDP. Due to economic meltdown and recession, a fall in GDP is imminent in the coming years, which may reduce CO_2 emission and result in a fall in global air pollution [17]. After the pandemic, air quality in many countries, including China, Italy, Spain, and the USA, has drastically improved. The apparent reason is a reduction in transportation and polluting industries. "These countries were also most affected by air pollution. The economic recession, linked to COVID-19, is likely to cause a drop in the carbon dioxide emissions for this year" [18].

On the contrary, the measures taken for controlling COVID-19 should not be mistaken for a long-term permanent solution to improve air quality. These measures are neither sustainable nor viable. A worldwide pandemic that is claiming human lives certainly should not be seen to bring about climate change. It is far from certain, for one thing, how lasting this plunge in emissions will be. After some time, when this pandemic finally subsides, will carbon dioxide and pollutant emissions bounce back, or could the changes we see now have a more permanent effect? [19] The answer is pending, even in the minds of world leaders. However, the probability of a bounce back with greater force is likely.

The primary cause of present and future climate change dynamics is human activities [20]. There are variations in local beliefs about this issue in the world. Some believe that it is a natural phenomenon, whereas the majority believe that human beings are the real cause of climate change; even industrial and transportation pollution are due to human beings, as they are the drivers behind them [21]. The belief in scientific findings and climate literacy can play a more effective role in controlling the man-made climate change, rather than controlling the man himself.

The Linkage between Climate & the Pandemic

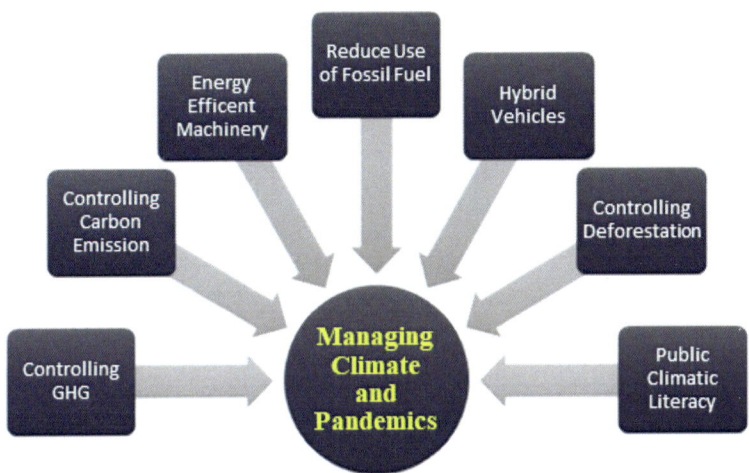

Figure 4.4: Managing Climate and pandemics.

Since every ounce of good has bad with it, and therefore bad too has some good, even if it may it be little in comparison. The pandemic has brought many ills, among other things, loss of a considerable number of human lives; the world has gone into a major recession after the great depression; and poverty and unemployment are likely to increase many fold, but the pandemic has so far had positive effects on the environment. The COVID-19 pandemic, to some extent, has an indirect relationship with climate change. The pandemic may, or may not, be the cause of environmental changes; it has yet to be confirmed, but contrary to the onslaught of the pandemic, the measures taken by states globally have had, overall, sound effects on the environment, as elucidated earlier. It is not yet scientifically determined whether both air quality and the spread of the present pandemic are linked, or are a coincidence. So far as the present pandemic and climate change are concerned, there is a clear and phenomenal link between the measures taken for control of the pandemic and the improvement of air quality, even if temporary.

In 2003, Epstein and colleagues at Harvard Medical School, in their study, deduced "human-induced changes in ecological systems and climate were triggering a barrage of emerging diseases that afflict humans, livestock, wildlife, marine organisms, and the very habitat we depend upon" [22]. It has been hypothesized that global climate change may cause pandemics in the future if viruses, presumably extinct, are released from the melting polar ice due to climate change. The same may result in extreme climatic change and a rise in sea levels. As human-induced systems trigger the climate and pandemics, literacy can also provide a vital tool in addressing them [23].

Climate change and other natural and artificial health problems affect human health and illnesses in several ways. These health problems are perpetual both in intensity and emergence. Day by day, the intensity of existing health problems will increase, and new health problems will be discovered. Everyone is at risk; pandemics and climate have no borders and are equally dangerous for human health and even lives [24].

"COVID-19 has demonstrated the interconnected nature of our world – and that no one is safe until everyone is safe" is a tweet from the official handle of the UN [25]. These pandemics, and climate change, affect both haves and have-nots. COVID-19 triggered enormous economic, emotional, mental, physical, and psychological suffering, and so does climate change, but at a slower speed. However, contrary to the above, another socialistic linkage at a deeper level exists, i.e., "Not everyone is equally at risk." Both climate change and pandemics differentiate between haves and have-nots. i.e., climate change is predominantly caused by richer countries as they are more industrialized. The poorer suffer the most in terms of flooding, homelessness, and the wide spread of diseases, etc. Similarly, the rich have accessibility to health facilities in global pandemics, while the poor do not. It is also sometimes referred to in the context of racism, wherein the white and yellow race is the major contributor of GHGs, but unfortunately, the brown and black have to bear the maximum burn.

Mother Earth is facing the existential challenges of the pandemic and climate change, and the entire race of homo sapiens is on the path to extinction. Unlike the dominating species of the past, humans themselves may be held responsible for their extinction. Similarly, although this world was not prepared to deal with pandemics unintentionally for climate change, the world is intentionally unprepared. Both climate change and the pandemic implicate market debacle, externalities, global collaboration, complex science, demands of system pliability, political determination, and timely action that centers on mass support. Significant state involvement is vital to stabilize the climate, by diverting energy and industrial systems towards innovative cleansers and a cost-effective means of production, and an effective and efficient global health system which responds to pandemics swiftly [26].

Both climate change and the pandemic have a linkage with health, but the former undermines the overall natural and human systems, whereas the latter threatens individuals and health systems. The response to COVID-19 demands quick and immediate actions, whereas the climate change response is less speedy and appears less acute. However, studies predict that climate change will deteriorate the longer we wait. Therefore, the crisis is overlapping and requires quick social awareness and mobilization. The devastating results of unprepared health systems, even those of the developed world after facing shocks like this pandemic, would realize the imprints of global environmental changes. Amongst these bearings on global health, some have a predominant environmental change signature, like the increasing range and spread of diseases such as malaria, dengue, COVID-19 pandemic. However, the relationship with climate change is less clear [27, 28]. The weakest link with COVID-19 in the global health chain threaten health everywhere of the evolving infectious diseases 70% are zoonotic [27, 28]. No one knows whether COVID-19 will be proven as a cause of climate change, or mingling in the natural cycle.

The world's efforts are presently focused on the COVID-19 pandemic. However, there seems to be a profound and worrying inter-relationship between this pandemic, climate changes, and decreased biodiversity, which needs urgent consideration. While the destruction of habitation, mainly by deforestation, is the core reason for diminishing biodiversity, another reason for the shift of habitat seems to be due to global environmental changes which compel living organisms. These organisms shift from one geographical range to another to survive and, ultimately, to get nearer to semi-natural habitats. In this way, these wild animals get closer to human habitats and livestock and carry in new microbes [29, 30].

Climate change is considered to be one of the significant reasons for communities' displacement. According to the UN Refugee Agency (UNHCR), out of 196 states affected by COVID-19 worldwide, 79 are hosting refugees that report the local spread of COVID-19 [29-31]. These communities are unavoidably spreading COVID-19. Experience with past epidemics and pandemics, i.e., Ebola, Severe Acute Respiratory Syndrome (SARS) and Middle East Respiratory Syndrome (MERS), gives us vital lessons in which to formulate policies for climate change as we find the way to deal with the challenges ahead [32]. The present pandemic provides a chance to understand, and to alleviate, upcoming disasters by diagnosing conceptual differences and connections between COVID-19 and global climate change.

Lessons Learnt from the Pandemic (COVID-19)

Every crisis brings an opportunity within itself. The COVID-19 pandemic has been declared a Public Health Emergency of International Concern (PHEIC), which has claimed hundreds of thousands of lives and is a major crisis globally. Therefore, there is a need to have a collective and global approach to deal with it, unlike the present crisis of climate change. There seems to be an entangled link between this pandemic and climate change, like another infectious disease that future research will unveil. Citizens across the globe should understand the effects of the pandemic and climate change on all of us. To address such problems in the future, a solution must be reached without compromising human life. The world must come out of profiteering capitalist business models where they compromise on the collateral damage of their industries, destroying the future of planet earth, reducing the period of human civilization, and paving the way for a more dangerous pandemic. It is akin to eating one's young [33].

Global health security requires an all-hazards approach to preparedness, from transmittable disease outbreaks to extreme weather events, to gradual climate change. Inequality is the main barrier to ensuring health and wellbeing, particularly for the most vulnerable in society. Estimates indicate that unnecessary environmental risks cause about one-fourth of global health problems. Early action protects the lives of human beings. A delay in the response to threats, whether from climate change or pandemics, increases the human and socioeconomic costs. If not addressed simultaneously, the environmental factors of health may inversely affect the response to COVID-19 due to the damages of climate change, and further burden health systems. The origin of recent infectious diseases, as elucidated earlier, is believed to be from wildlife. The evidence suggests that it is because of the human pressure on the natural environment that there is an emergence of new diseases. The protection of biodiversity may improve the health system [33].

The COVID-19 pandemic is linked to bats, but the response is superficial; the global community ignores the primary causes that may reduce the chances of an outbreak, if addressed timely. Controlling deforestation and wildlife habitats may significantly reduce the risk of future spreads [34]. We need to encourage afforestation and mobilize resources to spread awareness regarding its importance. Similarly, the deteriorating situation of air quality needs to be checked as it has been noted that air quality is significantly linked with the COVID-19 pandemic and could help contain COVID-19

[35]. Both scientific knowledge and facts matter in establishing a body of knowledge. Unfortunately, in both the COVID-19 and the environmental change scenarios, the growing scientific findings and facts derived on the same basis are being ignored. It is assumed that both hazards will vanish by themselves. This attitude will not save us from the unfolding grave consequences. These facts will chase us no matter whether we realize it or not. In regard to COVID-19, this realization is soon to come, whereas, with climate change it may take years. The sooner we realize it, the better it may be. In hindsight, we can analyze that at the start of COVID-19 the response of different nations was of denial mode. Interestingly, it resembles the six stages of climate denial mode, as shown in Figure 4.5.

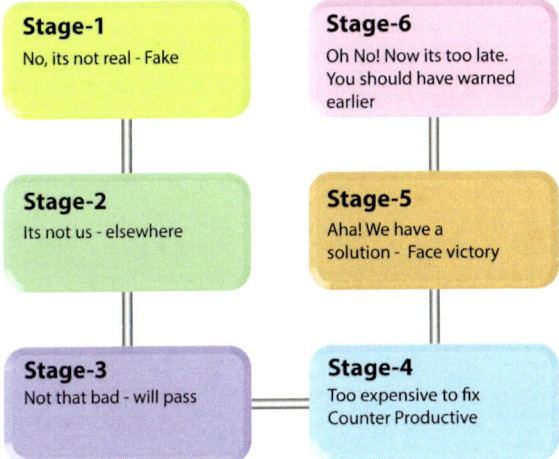

Figure 4.5: Stages of climate denial mode.

The COVID-19 crisis should be the turning point to believe in facts and the scientific body of knowledge. The health and wellbeing of human beings and their surroundings should be the priority while making decisions. "Making rational decisions based on the science and facts is our best weapon against our common enemies" [24] Lastly, such crises provide openings for a re-claimed intellect of collective humanity during which people recognize their health and safety, as a result of the extension of the health and safety of their surrounding community, and other global citizens. The pandemic and climate crisis threats relate us to one common goal of caring for each other and our environment. There is a need to have a global awareness campaign, including climate change literacy, effective media campaigns, and climate narrative building.

Conclusions

The world is now facing the biggest crisis of this generation. The decisions taken by individuals and governments will shape the world for the coming decades. They will change our health care systems and our societies, economies, politics, and culture. We should act more quickly and determinedly. The long-term consequences of our actions should also be taken into consideration. While choosing alternatively, we should ask ourselves how to overcome the instant threat, and what type of world we will make our home once the storm passes. The storm will pass, humankind will continue to exist, most of us will still be alive, but we will be in an entirely different world. Many immediate strategy measures will become a contest for our lives [39]. The world of climate change may suffer in the post-pandemic period for multiple reasons, including donors' policy priorities and funds, the viability and preferential treatment of climate change organizations, and the adoption of international laws and conventions regarding climate change. States will recover their economies as a top priority in which they may ignore pro-climate organizations, their funding, and its laws. However, all must realize that taking care of Mother Earth will reward us in the form of reduced risk of infectious diseases. This will guarantee the survival of the human race and have lasting effects on our progress and prosperity. Let us not forget that the next pandemic could be more lethal than this one. In the words of many academicians, the likely scenario for the cause of humanity's extinction lies with the effects of climate change or technological disaster.

Human causes of climate change significantly influence physical distancing after worldwide lockdown policies are enacted. Biological threats, deliberate or otherwise in any state, can threaten universal health, global security, and the international economy. Because communicable infections have no limits, all nations must prioritize and figure out the competencies required to avert, sense, and quickly react to public health emergencies. Every country should be clear about its know-how to guarantee neighbors that it can stop an epidemic from becoming a pandemic. Globalization has created numerous institutions that ensure the mobility of people, goods and services and, consequently, promote free trade. However, it has failed to develop everyday, collective rules for environmental standards, labor markets, health policy, and strategies for the emerging redistribution problems through standard social policy. In turn, world leaders and organizations owe a shared responsibility for developing and maintaining solid global competency to check communicable diseases and climate change. This competency comprises guaranteeing that funding is available to fill gaps in epidemic preparedness and climate change control. These measures will protect lives and lead to a safer and more secure world. Studies have concluded that early and timely climate change policies should be promoted to control the spread of infectious diseases such as COVID-19. Proactive instead of reactive policies need to be adopted. Individually and globally, we need to be countering the negative impacts of pandemics and climate change instead of firefighting.

References

1. Ruhl JB. Climate Change Adaptation and the Structural Transformation of Environmental Law. Environ Law. 2010; 40: 363.

2. Kahn, K., 2020. How scientists could stop the next pandemic before it starts. New York Times. Available at: https://www.nytimes.com/2020/04/21/magazine/pandemic-vaccine.html.

3. Hepburn C, O Callaghan B, Stern N, Stiglitz J, Zenghelis D. Will COVID-19 fiscal recovery packages accelerate or retard progress on climate change?. Oxford Review of Economic Policy. 2020; 36 (Supplement 1): S359-S381.

4. Kim R, Costello A, Campbell-Lendrum D. Climate change and health in Pacific island states. Bull World Health Organ. 2015; 93(12): 819. doi:10.2471/BLT.15.166199

5. Flannery TF. The weather makers: How man is changing the climate and what it means for life on earth. Grove Press, 2006; 18-22; 34-38.

6. Lia P. Can the pandemic sound the alarm on climate change? [online] Greenpeace International. Available at: https://www.greenpeace.org/international/story/29970/pandemic-alarm-climate-change-covid-19-coronavirus-environment/ [Accessed 3 Feb 2021].

7. Frumkin H, McMichael AJ. Climate change and public health: thinking, communicating, acting. American journal of preventive medicine, 2008; 35 (5): 403-410.

8. Chakraborty I, Maity P. COVID-19 outbreak: Migration, effects on society, global environment, and prevention. Science of the Total Environment, 2020; 728: 138882.

9. Lombrana, L.M. and Warren, H., 2020. A pandemic that cleared skies and halted cities isn't slowing global warming. Bloomberg Green. Available at: https://spotlightonpoverty.org/news/a-pandemic-that-cleared-skies-and-halted-cities-isnt-slowing-global-warming/ cited dated February 26, 2021.

10. McCollum D, Yang C, Yeh S, Ogden J. Deep greenhouse gas reduction scenarios for California–Strategic implications from the CA-TIMES energy-economic systems model. Energy Strategy Reviews. 2012; 1 (1): 19-32.

11. World-nuclear.org. (2019). Renewable Energy and Electricity | Sustainable Energy | Renewable Energy - World Nuclear Association. [online] Available at: https://www.world-nuclear.org/information-library/energy-and-the-environment/renewable-energy-and-electricity. aspx [Accessed 3 Feb. 2021].

12. Boden, T.A., G. Marland, and R.J. Andres. 2017. Global, Regional, and National Fossil-Fuel CO_2 Emissions. Carbon Dioxide Information Analysis Center, Oak Ridge National Laboratory, US Department of Energy, Oak Ridge, Tenn., USA doi 10.3334/CDIAC/00001_V2017

13. VOA (2020). Study: COVID-19 Shutdowns Cut Greenhouse Gas Emissions 17% | Voice of America - English. [online] www. voanews.com. Available at: https://www.voanews.com/covid-19-pandemic/study-covid-19-shutdowns-cut-greenhouse-gas-emissions-Emissions%2017%25 [Accessed June 3. 2020].

14. Chris Mooney, Chris Mooney, John Muyskens. Global emissions plunged an unprecedented 17 percent during the coronavirus pandemic. Available at: https://www.washingtonpost.com/climate-environment/2020/05/19/greenhouse-emissions-coronavirus/?arc404=true. Cited date February 26, 2021.

15. World Health Organization. Air pollution. Available at: https://www.who.int/news-room/air-pollution. Cited date February 26, 2021.

16. Meo SA, Suraya F. Effect of environmental air pollution on cardiovascular diseases. Eur Rev Med Pharmacol Sci. 2015 Dec;19(24):4890-7.

17. Wang H, Abajobir AA, Abate KH, Abbafati C, Abbas KM, Abd-Allah F, Abera SF, Abraha HN, Abu-Raddad LJ, Abu-Rmeileh NM and Adedeji IA. Global, regional, and national under-5 mortality, adult mortality, age-specific mortality, and life expectancy, 1970–2016: a systematic analysis for the Global Burden of Disease Study 2016. The Lancet, 2017; 390 (10100), 1084-1150.

18. Aristos Georgiou. Coronavirus Is Having a Major Impact on the Environment, With Reduced CO_2, Better Air Quality and Animals Roaming City Streets. https://www.newsweek.com/coronavirus-major-impact-environment-co2-air-quality-animals-1493812. Cited date February 26, 2021.

19. Gordon, J.T. (2020). The implications of the coronavirus crisis on the global energy sector and the environment. [online] Atlantic Council. Available at: https://www.atlanticcouncil.org/blogs/new-atlanticist/the-implications-of-the-coronavirus-crisis-on-the-global-energy-sector-and-the-environment/ [Accessed July 3. 2020]. Henriques, M., 2020.

20. Will Covid-19 have a lasting impact on the environment. BBC News, London, March 27.

21. Brzezinski A, Kecht V, Van Dijcke D, Wright AL. Belief in science influences physical distancing in response to covid-19 lockdown policies. The University of Chicago, Becker Friedman Institute for Economics Working Paper, 2020; 56.

22. Epstein PR, Chivian E, Frith K. Emerging diseases threaten conservation. Environ Health Perspect. 2003;111(10): A506-A507. doi:10.1289/ehp.111-a506.

23. Wyns A. How climate change and the coronavirus are linked. [online] World Economic Forum. Available at: https://www.weforum.org/agenda/2020/04/climate-change-coronavirus-linked 2020; [Accessed 3 May 2020].

24. Jin S. COVID-19, climate change, and renewable energy research: we are all in this together, and the time to act is now. ACS Energy Lett. 2020; 5: 1709-1711. doi.org/10.1021/acsenergylett.0c00910.

25. United Nation, Twitter Post, 2020. https://twitter.com/UN/status/1279445363682877442

26. Acemoglu D, Aghion P, Bursztyn L, Hemous D. The environment and directed technical change. American economic review, 2012; 1021): 131-66.

27. Rosenbloom, D. and Markard, J., 2020. A COVID-19 recovery for climate, 368(6490):447. doi:10.1126/science.abc4887.

28. Rahman, M. M., Bodrud-Doza, M., Shammi, M., Md Towfiqul Islam, A. R., & Moniruzzaman Khan, A. S. (2021). COVID-19 pandemic, dengue epidemic, and climate change vulnerability in Bangladesh: Scenario assessment for strategic management and policy implications. Environmental Research, 192, 110303. https://doi.org/10.1016/j.envres.2020.110303

29. Jones, K.E., Patel, N.G., Levy, M.A., Storeygard, A., Balk, D., Gittleman, J.L. and Daszak, P., 2008. Global trends in emerging infectious diseases. Nature, 451(7181), pp.990-993.

30. Lorentzen, H.F., Benfield, T., Stisen, S. and Rahbek, C., 2020. COVID-19 is possibly a consequence of the anthropogenic biodiversity crisis and climate changes. Dan Med J, 67(5), p.A205025.

31. San Lau, L., Samari, G., Moresky, R.T., Casey, S.E., Kachur, S.P., Roberts, L.F., and Zard, M., 2020. COVID-19 in humanitarian settings and lessons learned from past epidemics. Nature Medicine, 26(5), pp.647-648.

32. Stefan Gössling, Daniel Scott & C. Michael Hall (2021) Pandemics, tourism and global change: a rapid assessment of COVID-19, Journal of Sustainable Tourism, 29:1, 1-20, DOI: 10.1080/09669582.2020.1758708

33. World Health Organization. Climate Change and COVID-19. [online] www.who.int. Available at: https://www.who.int/news-room/q-a-detail/q-a-on-climate-change-and-covid-19 2020; [Accessed 4 Jun. 2020].

34. Meo SA, Abukhalaf AA, Alomar AA, Alessa OM, Sami W, Klonoff DC. Effect of environmental pollutants PM-2.5, carbon monoxide, and ozone on the incidence and mortality of SARS-COV-2 infection in ten wildfire-affected counties in California. Sci Total Environ. 2021; 25; 757: 143948. doi: 10.1016/j.scitotenv.2020.143948.

35. Bashir MF, Ma B, Komal B, Bashir MA, Tan D, Bashir M. Correlation between climate indicators and COVID-19 pandemic in New York, USA. Science of the Total Environment. 2020; 728: 138835.

COVID-19: The Emerging World Order and Global Approach

Chapter

05

Khalid Mahmood Shafi

Summary

The world has witnessed the spread of epidemics since the beginning of recorded history. However, when epidemics convert into pandemics, it has far-reaching and global implications on every sphere of life, including international power structures and world politics. This chapter looks into the present state of the global power structure. It analyzes the potential emergence of a new world order – while considering different factors, including social, economic, political, and international cooperation in the context of the prevailing pandemic. The analysis generates three different scenarios, especially concerning the length and impact of the duration of a pandemic on the global economy, and subsequent implications for the global power structure. The chapter concludes that the pathogen does not discriminate between the haves-and-have-nots and, thus, forms a basis for global cooperation to fight COVID-19.

Keywords: COVID-19, New World Order, Global Politics, Globalization

Introduction

Various viral infections have been threatening, evolving, and re-emerging to adversely affect the overall health and human approaches in the world order. Indeed, we have had hundreds of outbreaks in the last 30 years alone. The outbreak of H5N1 bird flu in 1997, the extreme acute respiratory syndrome (SARS) in 2002, the pandemic of H1N1 swine flu in 2009, the Middle East respiratory syndrome (MERS) in 2012, the Ebola virus in 2014, and the Zika virus in 2015 are notable examples [1].

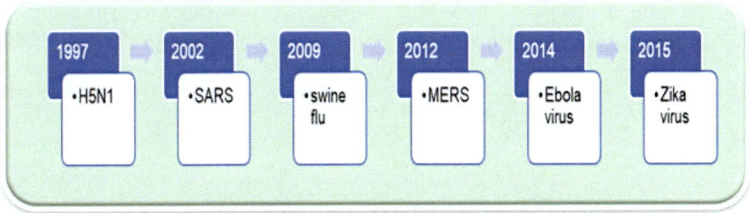

Figure 5.1: The emergence of epidemics/pandemics in the last 30 years.

Since December 2019, the novel coronavirus, Covid-19, has affected 207 countries and territories, infected 976,249 people with a mortality rate of 50,489 (5.17%) [2]. In the initial phase, China was the first to attempt to thwart and contain, while Italy and Iran followed; and despite the upperhand of prior warnings, all failed to restrict the virus. Other than the evident medical facilities and economic resources were the conceptual policy making and implementation. China, being a strict state, implemented measures aggressively and effectively. The military worked under government directives, and results were obtained. In Iran, the disconnection between the military and government officials was evident. In Iran, the advice of the military to restrict movement went unheeded, and later on, it was a disjointed and half-hearted effort [3].

On the other hand, Italy has a liberal democracy. When it tried to implement the isolation formula, it was defeated due to civic rights usurping slogans and a carefree attitude, until it was too late. The disastrous response of the USA served as an eye-opener to the limitations and exposed the policeman of the world. "Lessons were derived from World War I (1914-18) and World War II (1939-45), but what were the lessons from the threat, which affected a quarter of the world's population and the deaths of about 50 million in 1919?" Unfortunately, not much was derived from the Spanish flu; it was somewhat forgotten in the annals of history.

The Covid-19 pandemic created health, economic, political and social challenges, unseen and un-catered for worldwide. The Covid-19 pandemic revolutionized the global approach in interpreting the dimensions of the threat. Policymakers and strategists have debated traditional and non-traditional security threats, especially in the emerging world order, wherein the wideners have overtaken the traditionalists [4]. Traditional security threats revolved around violation of human rights through the act of terrorism, nuclear war, civil war, inter or intra-state wars, struggle for power maximization, and other state-centric threats. However, the non-traditional security threats encompassed poverty, hunger, epidemics, food security, climate change impacts, and other assorted challenges beyond the serious consideration of the international community, including leading global institutions like the United Nations and others. These were the primary settings of the world order in the pre-COVID environment.

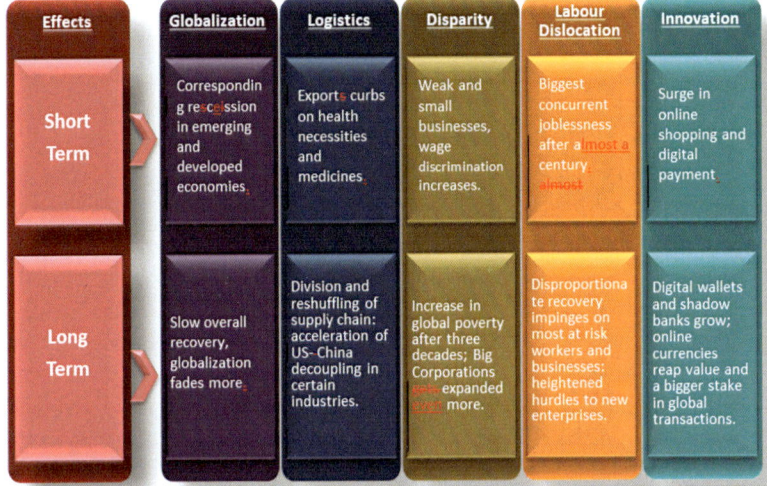

Effects	Globalization	Logistics	Disparity	Labour Dislocation	Innovation
Short Term	Corresponding recession in emerging and developed economies.	Exports curbs on health necessities and medicines.	Weak and small businesses, wage discrimination increases.	Biggest concurrent joblessness after almost a century almost	Surge in online shopping and digital payment.
Long Term	Slow overall recovery, globalization fades more.	Division and reshuffling of supply chain; acceleration of US–China decoupling in certain industries.	Increase in global poverty after three decades; Big Corporations gets expanded sizes more.	Disproportionate recovery impinges on most at risk workers and businesses; heightened hurdles to new enterprises.	Digital wallets and shadow banks grow; online currencies reap value and a bigger stake in global transactions.

Figure 5.2: Pandemic's effect on the economy

On the contrary, the greatest threat to the maintenance of global peace and security for human survival has emerged from this coronavirus pandemic, for which neither individuals nor nations were prepared. The causes and effects of this real threat have surpassed the heralds of nuclear war, terrorism, and even climate change. It has completely rearranged the world order and priorities.

Now, what miniscule lessons has the emerging pathogen taught us 7.8 billion humans at the start of the new decade, after all? Threats to humanity are not confined, and borders and financial situations limit neither. This crisis motivates us to see through the fog of fake individualism at the national and international levels. The role of institutions has been rearranged. The United Nations Security Council (UNSC) has been replaced by the World Health Organization (WHO). The medical fraternity has gained ancillary importance in collaboration with the military. Medical and paramedical workers are the new frontline soldiers. Netizens are the mouths and ears, which, with medical authentication can become credible and compelling. In dealing with any threat, the importance of planning and coordination is essential. What is required is to have a single-mindedness of conception at the highest levels, incorporating medical experts and harmonious execution at the lowest field levels. Fear-provoking pathogens, such as Covid-19, can be considered a revelation, turning the challenges into opportunities.

However, one thing is sure; that life will not be the same as in the pre-COVID era. A new world order is in the offing, mainly dictated by the global approach adopted in the post-COVID period

COVID-19 and the Outbreak

Viruses have trillions of varieties. They are the most abundant biological entities. They are found only within the cells of living organisms and are present in most of the planetary ecosystems. They are thought to have played an essential role in the evolutionary history of life. As Nasir et al. 2012 [5] states, "Viruses are intriguing biological entities that are borderline between inanimate and living matter. They often integrate into cellular genomes and massively enrich the genetic repository of numerous organisms, including animals, plants, and fungi. Viruses are believed to have played an important role in the evolution of cellular organisms" [5]. If one assesses, COVID-19 is an infectious disease on an unparalleled scale, caused by a newly discovered coronavirus. It belongs to the Coronavirus subgenus, a Betacoronavirus genus of the subfamily Orthocoronavirinae, in the family Corona viridae of the suborder cornidovirineae, of the order Nidovirales. It was later renamed SARS-CoV-2 by the International Committee on Taxonomy of Viruses. There are different opinions concerning its origin. Although initial studies reported a relation between a single local fish and the wild animal market, indicating possible animal-to-human transmission, now, studies have increasingly verified human-to-human transmission of SARS-CoV-2 through droplets or direct interaction. "A pestilence does not have human dimensions, so people tell themselves that it is unreal, that it is a bad dream that will end" [6].

This is not the first time that the human race has faced such a pandemic in the history of the disease. Medical history reveals that many epidemics or pandemics have taken thousands of human lives worldwide for centuries [7]. At the beginning of December 2019, the primary pneumonia cases of unidentified origin were found in Wuhan, the capital city of Hubei province [8]. The pathogen has been identified as a novel encased RNA beta coronavirus that has currently been named severe acute respiratory syndrome coronavirus 2 (SARS-CoV-2), which has a phylogenetic similarity to SARS-CoV [9]. Affected individuals were reported in family groups as well as hospital settings [10]. The virus has various biological, clinical, and epidemiological characteristics.

On January 30, 2020, ensuing the endorsements of the Emergency Committee, the WHO Director-General acknowledged that the outbreak constituted a Public Health Emergency of International Concern (PHEIC) [11]. The virus had almost engulfed the entire globe within four months and caused colossal damage to human lives, health, economies, industries, and other life activities (Figure 5.1) [12]. The world has been in a state of inertia, in so far as human activities are concerned.

Though it is a scientific issue, its effects have been felt across all walks of life. All nations are adversely affected, redefining state priorities in which an upcoming world order with changed priorities has emerged.

For leaders all over the world, the Covid-19 pandemic is a massive, universal examination. For all leaders, the problems posed were identical, but the policy solutions differed considerably. Just after the pandemic broke out, some regimes, like those of Australia or Argentina, implemented strict measures. In contrast, others like Brazil, Sweden, or the United States, opted for looser policies. In part, there are significant variations in the size and dynamics of infection rates, due to such diverse policy responses and their pacing. Initially, in March 2020, Europe saw a rapid rise in COVID case numbers, accompanied by a rapid fall. The United States and Brazil, on the other hand, continued to struggle [13].

World Politics and the Coronavirus Pandemic

The COVID-19 pandemic has immense historical importance, located at the confluence of two intertwined social dynamics – neoliberalism and the climate emergency – the disruptive existence of which causes the world to reconsider the structure of cultures, and our interaction with other human beings and the earth [14].

Politics has been suspended, societies are under lockdown, parliaments have closed, and a State of Emergency is in force globally [15]. "Epidemics, like disasters, have a way of revealing underlying truths about the societies they impact". They also reveal underlying truths about the relationship of a government and its citizens [16]. It seems as if world politics is in a state of pause, and suddenly, the priorities have changed and the challenges of a pandemic is the biggest priority of the time, for all states. Many on the European left, such as the Slovenian philosopher Slavoj Žižek, also fear an authoritarian contagion, predicting in the west "a new barbarism with a human face – ruthless survivalist measures enforced with regret and even sympathy, but legitimized by expert opinions" [17].

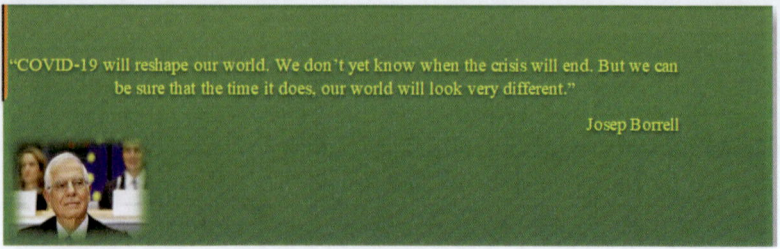

"COVID-19 will reshape our world. We don't yet know when the crisis will end. But we can be sure that the time it does, our world will look very different."

Josep Borrell

Unfortunately, the COVID-19 disease affects all aspects of human lives. Recently, some economic concerns, like the rising cases of unemployment, have raised serious questions about the lockdown strategy and how it could be carried out. Given the global socio-economic impact of COVID-19 on countries, governments should have an appropriate policy to help people by providing supportive materials, or loans, to compensate for any losses [18]. No differences exist in the capacity and capability of varying nations to offer support during the lockdowns.

As per Mr. Frankopan, two varying narratives can be perceived from COVID, collaboration and isolation. The interplay of collaboration and isolation is very intriguing. The time and space bondages of COVID-19 are also very interesting. The time was Brexit, Climate Change, and China and the USA in an emerging trade war. Space was COVID-19's initial emergence in China, followed by Iran, then spreading around Europe. The USA made unverified claims on COVID-19's emergence, spread, and the policies adopted in its aftermath, especially against China and the WHO. Historians have forewarned that the ordeal of a pandemic can be fertile ground for populist rhetoric rejoicing a mythical past [19, 20].

The New World Order

More than 50 million people worldwide were killed by the 1918 pandemic, popularly known as the Spanish flu, of which more than 14 million died in British India alone. The result of this pandemic has become far more profound and worldwide. World War I had a significant effect. It altered the borders of colonial powers and induced large-scale hardship in many countries, due to unemployment and inflation. In the former colonies, the pandemic reinforced independence struggles and pushed governments to develop policies for universal health care. It has also contributed to developments in epidemiology, virology, and vaccine production [20].

One aspect becomes apparent as countries firefight the Covid-19 pandemic;

the post-coronavirus planet will be different politically, socially, and health-wise in several respects. No one can come out of this situation without losing something [21]. The Covid-19 pandemic has escalated the debate among optimists, pessimists, and centrists about a paradigm shift in the world economic order. Although optimists anticipate the continuity of economic globalization after the pandemic, pessimists, considering the systemic negative effect of the pandemic on the world economy, predict localization instead of globalization. Conversely, the centrists expect a "U-shaped" rebound, where globalization will not be destroyed but slowed down by Covid-19. The three new viewpoints on the effect of Covid-19 on economic globalization are not without value, but they do not take an adequate temporary distance from the current problem [22].

The existing players were undermined by the chain of adverse outcomes of continual events. The economic power of the USA and Western countries is under debate. Their unchallenged dominance is being weakened. New players are developing and gaining popularity, such as China. China is second to the United States and has questioned the supremacy of the United States in the political, military, and economic spheres [23]. The United States has begun to feel the heat, and has initiated an all-out campaign to fight China via the use of negative propaganda instruments, the establishment of trade barriers, the introduction of technical growth restrictions, and the weakening of China's overall function.

Against the background of the pandemic, a new rivalry between the developed and the developing nations, if not a battle, is a unique and emerging phenomenon. Globalization's supporters and opponents are arguing for, and against, the doctrines of globalization. Emerging powers like China are now the system's proponents and are making every attempt to save it. The global political scenario has been complex, but exciting. Globalization is on trial, and the concept is being debated by almost every section of society. From ordinary citizens to academics and policymakers to the business community, everyone is guessing if globalization will survive the pandemic. It is then pertinent to ask the following questions:

Will there be a new world order after the pandemic? Will there be a shift in global power politics and existing power centers? The subsequent analysis will discuss and analyze these questions.

Suppose one assesses the primary effect of the post-COVID-19 pandemic. In that case, it is evident that from lifestyle to work ethics, in every aspect and way, an individual and organization are transformed according to COVID social norms.

"This much is certain: just as this disease has shattered lives, disrupted markets, and exposed the competence (or lack thereof) of governments, it will lead to permanent shifts in political and economic power in ways that will become apparent only later" [24].

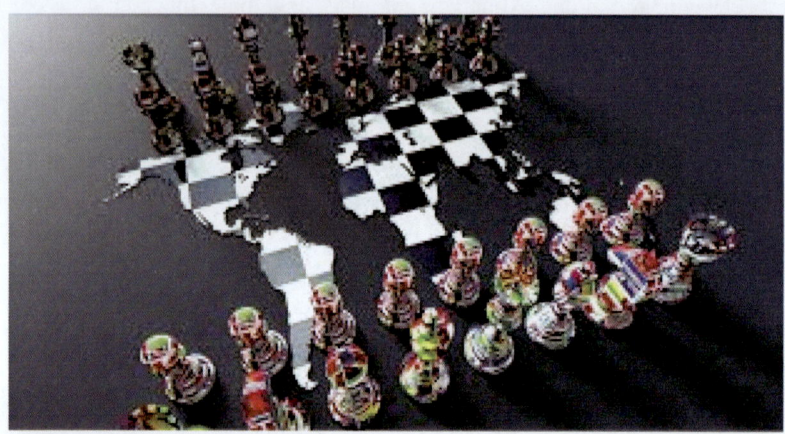

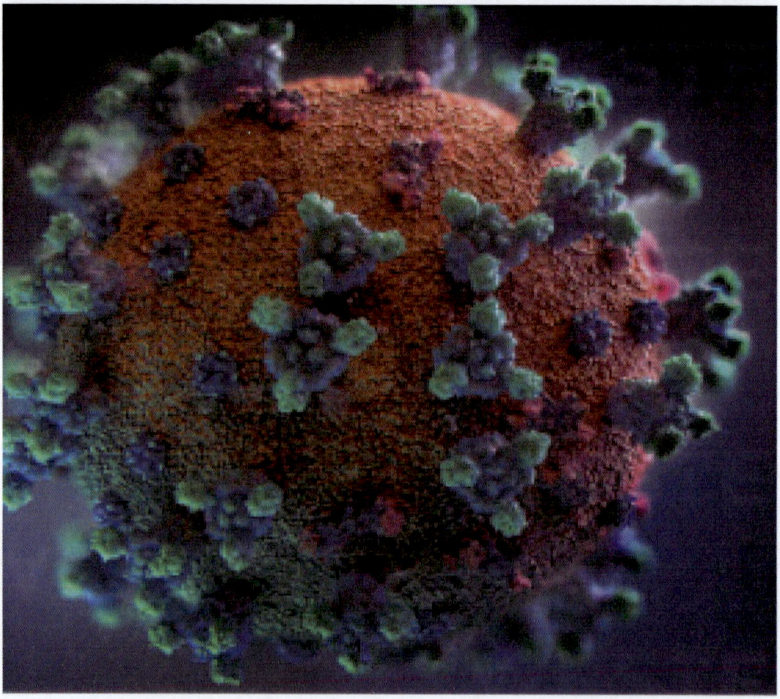

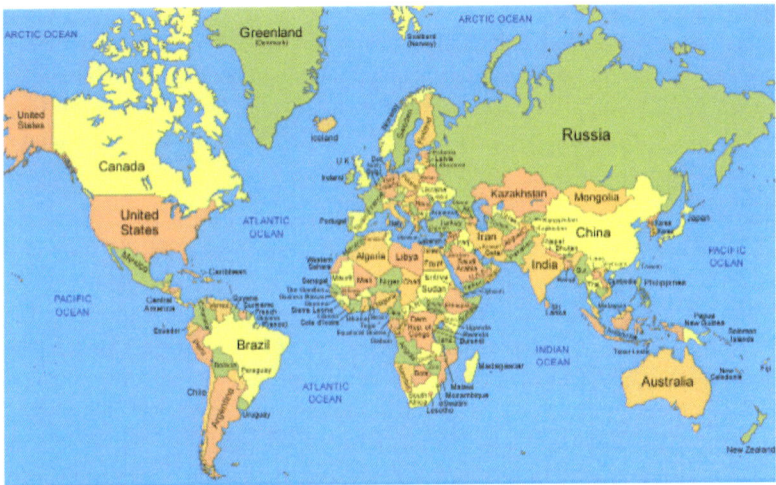

From the outset, the coronavirus pandemic has been a severe and massive shock to the post-World War II order, founded by the United States and its allies. For the past 75 years, the U.S. and its allies have been ruling the world based on liberal democratic principles, an inclusive global economy – and structured institutional bodies funded by strong democratic states. This order, though, has not gone unchallenged. Since then, Afghan wars and several other regional international conflicts have affected the global power trends, but the COVID-19 pandemic has threatened the survival of the entire global political order. The worsening state of Western economies has given China a much-awaited space in the world market economy. While a worldwide slump could spur protectionist support, China's economy has continued to grow, and its across continents' investments are staggering. Lateral bodies established to preserve public health become fragile and powerless to contain the problem, and as nations turn inward and close borders, alliances with transatlantic allies fray. A definitive global and US-led approach to the pandemic involves preserving and revitalizing the rule-based system that has ensured democracy, stability, and peace for decades [25].

The U.S. economic leadership has also been set at stake by the coronavirus pandemic. Countries are watching to see how fast the U.S. is getting past the crisis, whether it takes on the mantle of global leadership in response to the pandemic, and whether emerging economic superpowers, especially China, will more successfully weather the storm. Consequently, the global order could be radically reshaped by the virus, especially if the world's major economic powers, the United States, the European Union (E.U.), and China, experience widespread economic depression and restrict involvement outside their borders. If it is seen as being unable to handle the pandemic or unable to offer support to allies overseas, the United States could also face a significant drop in quiet strength [26]. Trump's isolationist policies have also acted as a catalyst to the fragile situation.

Both the United States and China need one another to ensure a chance for a global recovery in the immediate period. China reshaped the economy in 2008 and thereby enabled the rest of the world to rebound. However, it is uncertain if China today has the same power. The overall debt burden of China is nearly 310 percent, and several analysts suggest that it has little craving for a new economic incentive program. Protectionism and U.S.-China frictions will grow much more significant in this polluted environment if the world rebound is lengthy and sluggish and does not focus on employment; both of the current leaders in the United States and China will face actual checks. The fact of the matter is that, on the one hand, the coronavirus pandemic may end up strengthening the authoritarian instincts of Chinese President Xi Jinping and the Communist Party of China, and, on the other, an "America First" response.

A lack of European intergovernmental unity may cause more E.U. deterioration for the third time over the last decades (migration, the eurozone crisis, and now COVID-19). Traditionally, however, problems have driven the E.U. to greater integration. The virus has severely hit Europe, and a trend of individual efforts is on the rise, catalyzed by Brexit. Without U.S. aid and China's approval, Europe's prospects of saving the multilateral system for economic integration and foreign relations are very slim.

Considering the worst-case scenario, if the pandemic persists beyond a year or two, then a breakdown in the global socio-economic system is not an improbable scenario for Petro states from Ecuador to Iran. In the 1980s, though, Gorbachev's glasnost and perestroika initiated the disintegration of the Soviet Union; it was triggered by oil prices affecting the masses. There could be a similar situation for many Petro states. Venezuela's new years of hyperinflation and famishment will be compounded by trickling aid, and oil prices hitting rockbottom [27]. It may affect Middle East sources of revenue; oil and gas [28]. Iran's problems have been compounded by the stranglehold of American sanctions in the COVID environment. Developing and petrol-driven nations have been forced to approach the IMF to lease its emergency lending facility. They have also drawn down their dollar reserves to support their funding and stave off capital flight. Gulf states may need to release their U.S. dollar pegs [29]. The effect of the pandemic is exposing, once again, the risks of being too dependent on hydrocarbons for economic development, for the big oil and gas producing states. Global oil prices are currently floating between $20-$30 a barrel, and a deep global recession is looming, if not already here. Sustained low oil prices would mean this. How the diplomatic reshuffling of the area will be affected is less evident. Each of the regional forces faces its own internal (domestic), economic, and public health problems associated with the virus. Of these, the question of oil production, as mentioned above, faces both Saudi Arabia and Iran. While none of them can escape unfairly, Iran is arguably in a weaker place, due to the double effect of the current U.S. sanctions, which have impacted its capacity to export its oil (even at lower prices) and to repatriate foreign sales revenues [30].

Whether the state is suppressing the real numbers is questionable. However, some analysts claim that the Russian government does not realize the magnitude of the virus because the initial experiments were inaccurate, and few Russians were tested. Russian President Vladimir Putin has had to admit that there will be no vote on constitutional reforms in April, and he has recently had to postpone the big Victory Day parade [31].

COVID-19 is likely to shift the influence and power, shortly, from the erstwhile West to the East. Two nations that have responded most appropriately and can be viewed as role models are South Korea and Singapore. However, China has also recovered well after the initial setbacks, especially after learning from the situation in the USA. The USA and the bulk of Europe's response and reaction mechanisms have been inadequate and lacking an apt response, exposing its myth and aura of the anti-east brand [32].

The situation in the USA has amply demonstrated that military, economic and political power does not imply that it holds complete sway over internal security incidents. It has exposed the drawbacks of the American welfare and social state claims. Additionally, the erratic behavior of the leadership and measures as threatening, the WHO have further downed the image of the USA in the comity of nations.[33]

On the contrary, the South Korean philosopher Byung-Chula Han, in a significant paper in El Paris, argues that "China will now be able to sell its digital police state as a model of success against the pandemic. China will display the superiority of its system even more proudly." As per his reckoning, western voters in their respective democracies, engrossed in safety and community, might be keen to reduce and even sacrifice those liberties. What is freedom when one is forced to remain restricted to your own house in confinement?[34]

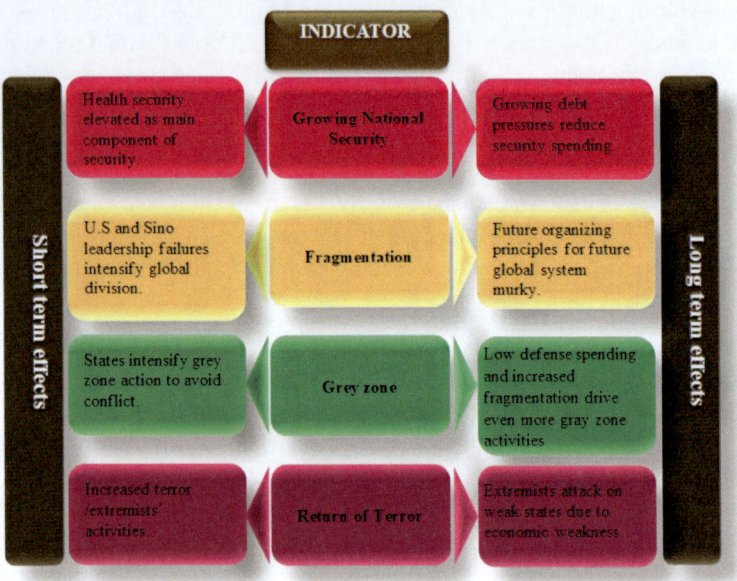

Figure 5.3: Implication of the Pandemic on Security.

Depending on the pandemic's disappearance, the ripple effects may not be as dreadful; some strong developed states may survive, but with less influence in world politics. Additionally, the country which resurrects itself from the impact of the pandemic will be automatically awarded the lead role. The pro pandemic economic acceleration would be helpful in this regard, among other economic indicators and factors. The economy will have to drive politics. Military might would be comparatively useless as the world would have gone through a catastrophe. However, the question is not of the world leader; the question is not race for dominance over the state nation being militarily powerful. These questions have miserably failed after the outbreak of the pandemic and its fast spread. The question would and should be "How could a nation keep its masses safe from an invisible, elusive enemy?" Previous plagues—counting the influenza epidemic of 1918-1919—utterly failed to lessen power rivalries, and they could not even enhance global cooperation, even in terms of medical sciences cooperation. Indeed, neither will COVID-19. It is predicted that there will be a further departure from hyper-globalization, as citizens look to governments to defend them and as states and firms seek to reduce imminent vulnerabilities [35]. What could be the possible political scenarios across the globe?

The Three Scenarios

The preceding discussion has been beautifully synthesized by Dr. Mathew J. Burrows, who serves as the director of the Atlantic Council's Foresight, Strategy, and Risks Initiative in the Scowcroft Center for Strategy and Security, in three scenarios:

1. Great acceleration downwards

2. China first

3. New renaissance.

Despite substantial fiscal and monetary initiatives, the American government, Europe, and China fail to recover. The rebound continues deep into the 2020s, compounded by the fact that it takes even longer than anticipated to produce a vaccine. Initially, plans were made to recreate the post-2008-09 financial crisis period with summits of G7 and G20 leaders to plan out a global recovery [36]. However, those summits quickly break down, and the regular blame game is restored to Washington and Beijing. A newly elected administration tries to take advantage of the crisis by seeking to wring concessions out of China to end state subsidies to state-owned enterprises (SOEs), to gain more market access for U.S. businesses, and protections for U.S. companies doing business in China against forced intellectual property tech transfers [37]. The United States imposes tariffs on Chinese exports and prohibits new Chinese investments as long as China refuses. For their part, Chinese leaders would try to stop introducing a massive stimulus package to the debt load, the way they did during the financial crash of 2008. Stimulus efforts by China are smaller in size [38].

The Netherlands, Germany, and the other northern E.U. members are pitched against the others. Germany is suspicious of the others making use of the crisis as a precedent for mutualizing peril across the E.U. The institutions of the E.U. are paralyzed while dissections deepen between the north and south. In evaluation, in its "decoupling" threats against China, Europe is torn about whether to back the United States. Many Europeans, and also U.S. public opinion, blames China for the pandemic. However, a growing number of countries in the south and east are thankful for Chinese assistance during the crisis, and much later, when new Chinese investments are being made in those areas.

Deglobalization is accelerating in the mid-2020s, yielding sluggish economic growth everywhere. Due to COVID-19, poverty levels are increasing in the developed world, and there is the possibility of an open confrontation between the United States and the China-Russia alliance.

Although China is the prime nation responsible for the outbreak, the pandemic has sloped the geopolitical balance in its favor. China has not entirely recovered, but its government sees a chance to weaken the legitimacy of Western liberal democracy by extending aid with expanded soft loans and other development programs. "Belt and Brace-type" agreements have been spread to more countries in Asia, Africa, and Latin America, granting Beijing control of vital infrastructures in more countries. At home, by presenting Western democracies as helpless to cope adequately with the pandemic, the CPC is actively strengthening popular support. For the many nations outside Europe, the USA appears to be in sharp decline.

As the global economy crashes, the heads of the G7 and G20 summits rise above populist instincts with a new U.S. leader at the helm and forge a consensus on a concerted recovery strategy, including removing border closures and loosening tariffs and other trade barriers. The recovery is gaining momentum after a slow start, and the major economies are seeing renewed progress. The V-shaped regeneration ultimately emerges. It took a year, though, before the take-off took place, assisted by the discovery and quick distribution of a vaccine. With the elimination of inter-state tensions, global prosperity is resuming, and the Sustainable Development Targets of reducing hunger and spreading education are once again within reach for the bulk of the world's population.

There will be a more optimistic shift in the definition of national interests in the post-pandemic era. It would be a more social welfare-based definition, rather than the existing one of acquiring power to surpass other states. There would be more stress and funding for the health and medical sectors. These priorities should emerge; if they don't, we humans would assert and prove the pessimistic approach towards human nature.

Global Approach

Globalization has led to a new generation of global people in recent decades. Although rights to this worldwide citizenship have not yet been evenly dispersed, millions have enjoyed unrestricted freedom to travel, work, and fly. However, COVID-19 has significantly slowed down this cosmopolitan globalization discourse about a borderless nation [39]. Several observers have noted that a global surge of nationalism may result from the pandemic and states' reactions as the world appeared to come to a standstill. The response continues to make nationalism more popular, from the closing of borders and the challenge of mobilizing support and unity around them to the insecurity many people feel as people look to support their groups [40]. It is far from clear whether what others have termed "*coronationalism*" or universal unity will challenge the world. It is both enticing and daunting to fortify the post-pandemic environment. Instead of accurate predictors, initial responses and the crisis climate can prove to be inaccurate or transient indicators. During the pandemic reaction, however, nationalism has been evident in various ways. This is no surprise, considering the increased significance of exclusionary nationalism before the pandemic, in multiple cultures and political debates worldwide. It also deserves reflection on how nationalism in the world is likely to be influenced by both the pandemic itself and the responses of various governments [41].

The world is facing one of its most significant global health problems. Coronavirus 2019 has shown how precarious our preparedness for global infectious disease is. With a fast travel time between its distant parts, the planet is a small-connected globe. COVID-19 has grown internationally and exponentially, with significant effects on population health, the economy, and the quality of life [42].

No one is safe. No village, no town, no city, no country, and no continents are safe. The other planets concerned are safe so far, due to the non-reach of human beings. We, human beings, carried it from animals and moved it to human beings. In a war of survival of the fittest, it is between human beings and a tiny virus. It is not the survival of the most appropriate nation-states. It is a war of survival of human beings. This virus has exposed the progress and development of human beings, the shallowness of the body of knowledge, the nature of human beings, and the real threats to the human race.

The less-developed times of the past were better. As far as the spread of a virus is concerned, it took years, but in the present-day, so-called, global village, it took days to spread all over the world. We intentionally, or unintentionally, ignored the invisible enemies of human beings and instead exhausted our energies on political enemies as our predecessors did in the past. We progressed technologically in our view, we saved ourselves from each other, but we ignored the real enemies of human beings, that exist in nature in their trillions. Paradoxically, globalization has facilitated the virus blowout like a wildfire across the globe. Modern modes of transportation have contributed to its spread. There is no denying that while science has the supremacy to nurture, it also influences destruction [43].

Addressing the nation on March 17, French President Emmanuel Macron declared "*nous sommes en Guerre*" (We are at war) adding: "The enemy is there invisible, elusive and it is advancing." Many other politicians have also taken to describing their country as being "at war" [44].

The world is not in a state of conflict because the pandemic we are confronting requires procedures that are, instead, the opposite of those adopted in wartime: scaling down economic bustle rather than enhancing it up, forcing a sufficient proportion of workers to time-out rather than mobilizing them to energize a war effort, radically dropping social interaction rather than sending all the services to the frontline. To say it candidly, let us put it this way: staying restricted to one's domestic premises, in the kitchen or bedroom, has no link with a period of conflict where one has to guard oneself against bombs and marksmen, and try to endure in exposed conditions [45].

For several years, the coronavirus pandemic that has rocked the planet would cast a long shadow. It places society in the face of enormous obstacles that overlap with other negative mega-trends and technological, social, and political issues that have not been addressed. The immense implications and costs of human and societal, economic, and financial pandemic treatment can only be understood ex-post. Although some risk nothing, others risk their lives, or lose everything. A diverse, post-pandemic future in which various political and economic regimes can engage with each other under conditions of irreversible globalization will take several directions, with the role of highly developed nations being comparatively weaker. Tensions will escalate on the US-China side, and geopolitics and geo-economics will change. The conflict between liberalism and authoritarianism will escalate, and the synergies between the economy and the state will change. The two sides of the same counterfeit coin would be particularly risky as an alternative: capitalist capitalism versus nationalist capitalism. A gradual shift to a new pragmatism will build prospects for a better future. It is a policy focused on a revolutionary, unorthodox, and systemic economic theory of moderation in economic practices and triple-economic, social, and ecologically sustainable growth. Pandemics are also a significant problem for social sciences, not just for economics, but old methods of reasoning are always obsolete for modern circumstances to be studied and explained.

References

1. Khan, G., Sheek-Hussein, M., Al Suwaidi, A.R., Idris, K. and Abu-Zidan, F.M., 2020. Novel coronavirus pandemic: A global health threat. Turkish Journal of emergency medicine, 20(2), p.55.

2. World Health Organization (2020). Coronavirus disease (COVID-19) pandemic. [online] Who.int. Available at: https://www.who.int/emergencies/diseases/novel-coronavirus-2019 [Accessed January 30 2021].

3. Peters, M.A., Jandrić, P. and McLaren, P., 2020. Viral modernity? Epidemics, infodemics, and the 'bioinformational'paradigm.

4. Sreenivas, n., is chakarpani, and p. Anil Kumar. "the paradigm of entry into host-concerns in developing antivirals for covid-19."

5. Nasir, A., Kim, K.M. and Caetano-Anollés, G., 2012. Viral evolution: primordial cellular origins and late adaptation to parasitism. Mobile Genetic Elements, 2(5), pp.247-252.

6. Camus, A., 2012. The plague. Vintage. https://www.amazon.com/Plague-Vintage-International-Albert-Camus-ebook/dp/B008QLVNII. Cited date February 23, 2021

7. Liyanage, S., Corona: Performativity of A Pandemic. https://www.colombotelegraph.com/index.php/corona-performativity-of-a-pandemic/Cited date February 23, 2012.

8. Huang, C., Wang, Y., Li, X., Ren, L., Zhao, J., Hu, Y., Zhang, L., Fan, G., Xu, J., Gu, X., and Cheng, Z., 2020. Clinical features of patients infected with 2019 novel coronavirus in Wuhan, China. The lancet, 395(10223), pp.497-506.

9. Lu, R., Zhao, X., Li, J., Niu, P., Yang, B., Wu, H., Wang, W., Song, H., Huang, B., Zhu, N. and Bi, Y., 2020. Genomic characterization and epidemiology of 2019 novel coronavirus: implications for virus origins and receptor binding. The lancet, 395(10224), pp.565-574.

10. Guan, W.J., Ni, Z.Y., Hu, Y., Liang, W.H., Ou, C.Q., He, J.X., Liu, L., Shan, H., Lei, C.L., Hui, D.S. and Du, B., 2020. Clinical characteristics of coronavirus disease 2019 in China. New England journal of medicine, 382(18), pp.1708-1720.

11. Meo SA, Al-Khlaiwi T, Usmani AM, Meo AS, Klonoff DC, Hoang TD. Biological and epidemiological trends in the prevalence and mortality due to outbreaks of novel coronavirus COVID-19. J King Saud Univ Sci. 2020 Jun;32(4):2495-2499. doi: 10.1016/j.jksus.2020.04.004. Epub 2020 April 9.

12. World Health Organization (2020). Coronavirus disease (COVID-19) pandemic. [online] Who.int. Available at: https://www.who.int/ emergencies/diseases/novel-coronavirus-2019 [Accessed January 30 2021].

13. Herrera, H., Ordoñez, G., Konradt, M., and Trebesch, C., 2020. Corona Politics: The cost of mismanaging pandemics.

14. Nunes, J., 2020. The COVID-19 pandemic: securitization, neoliberal crisis, and global vulnerabilization. Cadernos de saude publica, 36, p.e00063120.

15. Chandler, D., 2020. The Coronavirus: Biopolitics and the rise of 'Anthropocene Authoritarianism'. Russia in Global Affairs.

16. Wintour, P., 2020. Coronavirus: Who Will be winners and losers in the new world order. The Guardian.

17. Nourizadeh, M., Rasaee, M.J. and Moin, M., 2020. COVID-19 pandemic: A big challenge in Iran and the world. Iranian Journal of Allergy, Asthma, and Immunology.

18. Frankopan, P., 2017. These Days, All Roads Lead To Beijing. New Perspectives Quarterly, 34(4), pp.6-15.

19. Sharfuddin, S., 2020. The world after Covid-19. The Round Table, 109(3), pp.247-257.

20. WHO–UNICEF– Lancet Commissioners. After COVID-19, a future for the world's children? Lancet. 2020 Aug 1;396(10247):298-300. doi: 10.1016/S0140-6736(20)31481-1.

21. Wang, Z. and Sun, Z., 2020. From globalization to regionalization: The United States, China, and the post-Covid-19 world economic order. Journal of Chinese Political Science, pp.1-19.

22. Ramay, S.A., 2020. 21st Century global Order: Factors Behind Change.

23. Allen, J., Burns, N., Garrett, L., Haass, R.N., Ikenberry, G.J., Mahbubani, K., Menon, S., Niblett, R., Nye Jr, J.S., O'neil, S.K. and Schake, K., 2020. How the world will look after the coronavirus pandemic. Foreign Policy, 20, p.2020.

24. Burrows, J.M. and Engelke, P., 2020. What world post-COVID-19. Three Scenarios, Atlantic Council Strategy Papers.

25. Grint K. Leadership, management, and command in the time of the coronavirus. Leadership. 2020;16(3):314-319. doi:10.1177/1742715020922445

26. Spector B. Even in a global pandemic, there is no such thing as a crisis. Leadership. 2020;16(3):303-313. doi:10.1177/1742715020927111

27. Khanna, P. (2020). Six predictions for new world order – Virtual Speakers | Book Virtual Keynote Speakers. [online] www.virtualspeakers.com. Available at: https://www.virtualspeakers.com/virtual-speakers-blog/parag-khanna-coronavirus-butterfly-effect/ [Accessed January 29 2021].

28. Michelle Carmody. Available at: https://theconversation.com/what-caused-hyperinflation-in-venezuela-a-rare-blend-of-public-ineptitude-and-private-enterprise-102483. Cited date February 22, 2021.

29. Claudia Carpenter. https://www.spglobal.com/platts/en/market-insights/latest-news/oil/101920-oil-exporters-to-be-hurt-most-in-middle-east-by-coronavirus-imf. Cited date February 22, 2021.

30. Atlantic Council (2020). What world post-COVID. [online] Issuu. Available at: https://issuu.com/atlanticcouncil/docs/what_world_post_covid_final_042220 [Accessed January 29 2021].

31. Roth, A. (2020). Russia defies calls to halt Victory Day parade rehearsals. The Guardian. [online] April 6. Available at: https://www.theguardian.com/world/2020/apr/06/russia-defies-calls-to-halt-victory-day-parade-rehearsals [Accessed January 29 2021].

32. Allen, J., Burns, N., Garrett, L., Haass, R.N., Ikenberry, G.J., Mahbubani, K., Menon, S., Niblett, R., Nye Jr, J.S., O'neil, S.K. and Schake, K., 2020. How the world will look after the coronavirus pandemic. Foreign Policy, 20, p.2020."

33. Güler, M.A. (2020). The new world order with new values. [online] Daily Sabah. Available at: https://www.dailysabah.com/opinion/op-ed/the-new-world-order-with-new-values [Accessed January 30 2021].

34. Editor, P.W.D. (2020). Coronavirus: who will be winners and losers in the new world order? The Guardian. [online] April 11. Available at: https://www.theguardian.com/world/2020/apr/11/coronavirus-who-will-be-winners-and-losers-in-new-world-order [Accessed January 30 2021].

35. Allen, J., Burns, N., Garrett, L., Haass, R.N., Ikenberry, G.J., Mahbubani, K., Menon, S., Niblett, R., Nye Jr, J.S., O'neil, S.K. and Schake, K., 2020. How the world will look after the coronavirus pandemic. Foreign Policy, 20, p.2020."

36. BURROWS, M. and ENGELKE, P. (2020). What World POST-COVID-19?: Three Scenarios. [online] JSTOR. Available at: https://www.jstor.org/stable/resrep24634 [Accessed January 29 2021].

37. Qin, Julia Ya, Forced Technology Transfer, and the US-China Trade War: Implications for International Economic Law 2019; 61: https://ssrn.com/abstract=3436974 or http://dx.doi.org/10.2139/ssrn.3436974

38. Alexander Chipman Koty. https://www.china-briefing.com/news/chinas-stimulus-measures-after-covid-19-different-from-2008-financial-crisis/ cited date February 22, 2021.

39. Calzada, I. Platform and Data Co-Operatives amidst European Pandemic Citizenship. Sustainability, 2020; 12(20): 8309.

40. Bieber, F., 2020. Global nationalism in times of the COVID-19 pandemic. Nationalities Papers, 2020; 1-13.

41. Bieber, Florian. Debating Nationalism: The Global Spread of Nations. London: Bloomsbury, 2020.

42. Khan G, Sheek-Hussein, M., Al Suwaidi, A.R., Idris, K. and Abu-Zidan, F.M., 2020. Novel coronavirus pandemic: A global health threat. Turkish Journal of emergency medicine, 2020; 20(2): 55.

43. Mutlaq, A. (2020). Hoping for new world order after the coronavirus crisis. [online] Arab News. Available at: https://www.arabnews.com/node/1657731/hoping-new-world-order-after-coronavirus-crisis [Accessed January 30 2021].

44. Lal, V. (2020). The Coronavirus, the Enemy, and Nationalism. [online] Lal Salaam: A Blog by Vinay Lal. Available at: https://vinaylal.wordpress.com/2020/03/21/the-coronavirus-the-enemy-and-nationalism/ [Accessed January 30 2021].

45. Kolodko, G.W., 2020. After. Economics and politics of the post-pandemic world. Voprosy Ekonomiki, (5), pp.25-44.

Global Warming Pre- and Post- COVID-19 Pandemic

Chapter 06

Anusha Sultan Meo

Abstract

Besides the solutions mentioned in this chapter, learning a lesson from this COVID-19 pandemic is essential. The global community must think about how we lacked, where we lacked, and what steps we can take to avoid such a calamity, and so much loss of life, in the future. We have watched how helpless humanity is in front of the Divine Decree. Hence, if society cannot think, reflect and take heed from so much suffering over the past year, then perhaps nothing can change us. Maybe together, however, step by step, we can have hope that someday our targets can be met, and our dreams can be achieved. Thus, maybe shortly, we can hope that we head towards recovery; that life on this planet can go back to being as peaceful as our ancestors once was

Keywords: COVID-19 Pandemic, Global Warming, Pre- and Post-Pandemic

COVID-19: An insight

When the first case of the novel coronavirus, severe acute respiratory syndrome coronavirus-2 (SARS-CoV-2), COVID-19 pandemic, emerged on December 31, 2019, in a local food market of China, the world was not in the slightest prepared for mass mayhem in the form of what was to become a global pandemic. Initially misunderstood as mysterious cases of pneumonia, the World Health Organization reported on social media on January 4, 2020, that there was a cluster of pneumonia cases, with no deaths, however, in the Wuhan, Hubei province. A day later, these cases were recognized, and the WHO published their first Disease Outbreak News on the new SARS-CoV-2 virus. On January 13, fear began to rise globally as the alarming news broke out that the first case of this new virus was detected outside China, in Thailand. With a statement being issued of the evidence of human-to-human transmission of this new virus on January 22, the highly contagious virus involved the entire world; finally, the WHO, on March 11, 2020, declared this disease as a global pandemic.

As revealed by the statistics of January 8, 2021, the current number of coronavirus cases is 89,060,618, including 23,279,576 active cases and a total of 1,915,917 deaths since the beginning [2]. A year after the emergence of this disease, it was in December 2020, when the first ray of hope against the coronavirus surfaced, as the Pfizer and Moderna Vaccines [3].

Having undergone significant testing, these vaccines have been declared satisfactorily effective against the virus, mainly against the old strain, while testing their effectiveness against the new strains that emerged, mainly from the United Kingdom, continues. A year into this transformation of everyday life, we have seen how the pandemic has affected the global community, making every person adapt to living with masks, social distancing, and other suggested preventive measures. While strict rules are still being implemented in countries where COVID-19 is on the rise with a second or third wave, such as the United States or the United Kingdom, all countries, including those making their way back to normality, continue to impose safety restrictions on their citizens for the sake of their health, fearing the morbidity and mortality that this virus brought across the globe. The battle against the virus continues with physicians and health care workers at the frontline, sacrificing their well-being for individuals who have succumbed to this deadly disease, and yet despite all the precautions taken, Covid-19 has just recently found its way to the least inhabited continent in the world, Antarctica [4].

Given the numbers and the pandemic curve, such as those demonstrated by Figure 6.1, (data obtained from the Worldometer website) [5], we cannot deny the disastrous impact of COVID-19 on the human population's health care systems and giant economies. However, besides human beings, everything else on the planet has also been affected. This includes the environment surrounding us, nature, and our climate, which shall be discussed in the upcoming sections. It is well acknowledged that surroundings and weather conditions are highly essential and impact health and disease patterns.

Cumulative number of cases (by number of days since 10,000 cases)

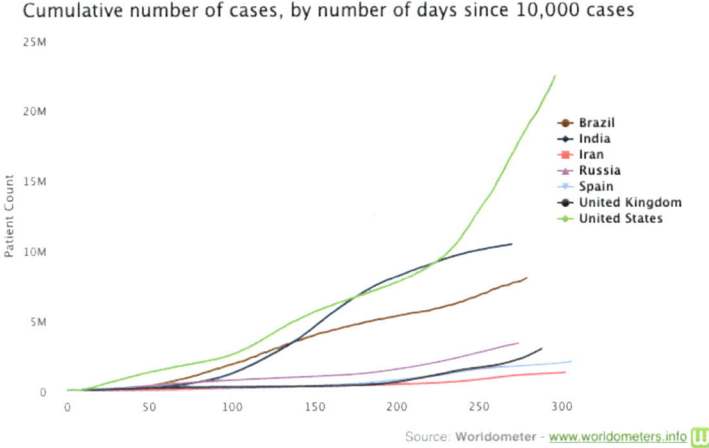

Figure 6.1: COVID-19 pandemic curve, for the cumulative number of cases (by number of days since 10,000 cases) source: https://www.worldometers.info/ [5]

The History and Phenomenon of Climate Change and Global Warming

Science has significantly expanded its research in all branches. Over many years, textbooks, the mass media, and the international scientific community have been emphasizing another global issue that is no less than a disease; this one, however, particularly deteriorating the health, not of people, but of the earth and, specifically, its climate. Climate change, which is the significant gradual drift in the pattern of global temperatures and rainfall, was discovered in the 19th century. The patterns of weather change were noticed when ice ages and other natural changes in paleoclimate were first suspected [6], owing to studies revealing that the earth's average temperature has increased by about 1.1°C since preindustrial times (1850-1900) [7].

An average warming, worldwide, of 1.1°C seems negligible. However, the dramatic effects this temperature rise produces on the whole, in different areas, are astounding. While some countries have experienced more significant changes in their weather patterns and witnessed a more significant increase in local temperatures, there is no denying that the consequences of melting glaciers in the Arctic and Antarctica resulting in rising sea levels, and unprecedented heatwaves in some areas, are proof of the damage that human beings have caused to the ecosystem; the culprit of climate change mainly being the increased emissions of gases from factories after the industrial revolution. Besides this, the usage of cars and other machinery that involve the release of toxic gases, and all other human activities resulting in air pollution, alongside the destruction of nature such as deforestation, contribute to this phenomenon as a whole. Due to all of the above activities, this increase in the average global temperature is termed global warming.

Recent studies conducted by the meteorological departments in different parts of the globe have predicted the following changes in the weather pattern, all resultant factors of global warming:

Heatwaves are becoming more common and severe. Evidence has been provided because records reveal that July, 2019 was declared the hottest month on earth since records started in 1880 [8]. These temperature rises, proving the impact of global warming, contribute to the further melting of ice caps and glaciers, accelerating other elements of climate change such as "rising sea levels." Droughts worldwide have increased in frequency and severity and are predicted to worsen over the years. This will eventually lead to a water crisis and food shortage in the suffering countries.

There has been an average global sea-level rise of 5 mm per year in the past five years. In time, this minor effect shall prove to have a catastrophic effect, e.g., in the form of mass flooding. Between 2007-2009, 2.5 million people lost their homes due to flooding as a consequence of sea-level rise. Just 0.5 meters of total sea-level rise would affect 800 million people living in 570 coastal cities worldwide by 2050, as portrayed by Figure 6.2, where the map shows cities with 10 million inhabitants, or more [9].

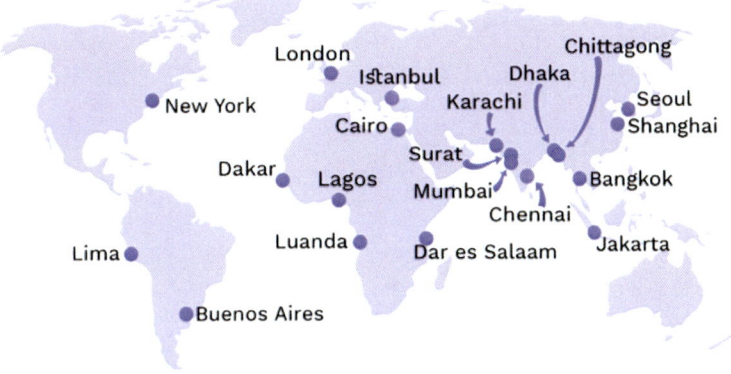

Cities at risk of 0.5m flooding in 2050
With 10,000,000+ people

Figure 6.2: Cities at risk due to coastal flooding [9].

Changes in forms of precipitation, such as rainfall and snowfall, shall be witnessed. Rainfall is much more difficult to predict than temperature, but there are some statements that scientists can make with confidence about the future [10]. With the given increases in temperature, a warmer atmosphere can hold more moisture, and globally water vapor increases by 7% for every degree centigrade of warming. This will translate into changes in global precipitation that is less clear-cut, but the total volume of precipitation is likely to increase by 1-2% per degree of warming. Different climate models reveal various expected changes; however, with growing expenditure on technological weather monitoring systems, these models are expected to improve and give us more reliable predictions and results. Evidence also shows that areas experiencing more significant precipitation will share more, and dryer areas witness less, thereby pushing the precipitation patterns to an extreme. Other observed and predicted consequences of global warming include the following, which have also been displayed in Figure 6.3:

Table 6.1: Predicted consequences of global warming.

- Flooding
- Decreased crop yields
- Food shortage
- Water crisis
- Vector-borne diseases
- Extreme rainfall
- Tropical cyclones
- Wildfires
- Cold events
- Loss of biodiversity
- Human migration
- Residential crisis
- Ocean acidification due to absorption of carbon emissions
- Coral reefs
- Extinction of animal species
- Economic collapse

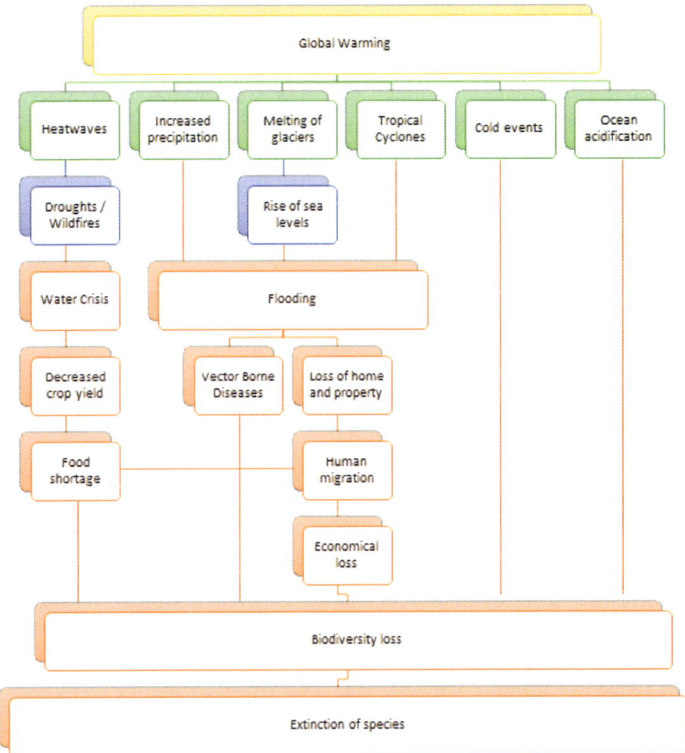

Figure 6.3: The diverse consequences of global warming and their impact on the ecosystem.

The various elements of nature and the ecosystem that are being disturbed by global warming will continue to deteriorate at accelerating rates in the future, rendering adverse effects not just on the planet, but significantly more on human life. Nevertheless, to bring a halt to climate change, we must ask ourselves the reasons why it is happening in the first place, by pondering over "what exactly is causing global warming and climate change?" This is where the Greenhouse Effect, discussed in the upcoming section, comes into play.

The Greenhouse Effect

Despite the tremendous amount of scientific evidence revolving around global warming and the establishment of international organizations such as the World Meteorological Organization, designated especially for research on this cause, a group of environmentalists and scientists still believe that global warming is a phenomenon not related to human activities, such as industrialization, but instead results from natural volcanic activity or solar variation. However, a correlation was seen between the temperature rise and degree of industrialization over the years, as shown by Figure 6.4 [11], and along with detailed studies of climate computer models and emphasis on the Milankovitch theory [12], it is becoming more evident that this effect was most likely due to the gases being released into the atmosphere from factories. The increasing concentration, above normal, of these gases in the atmosphere is causing the shift in the global climate.

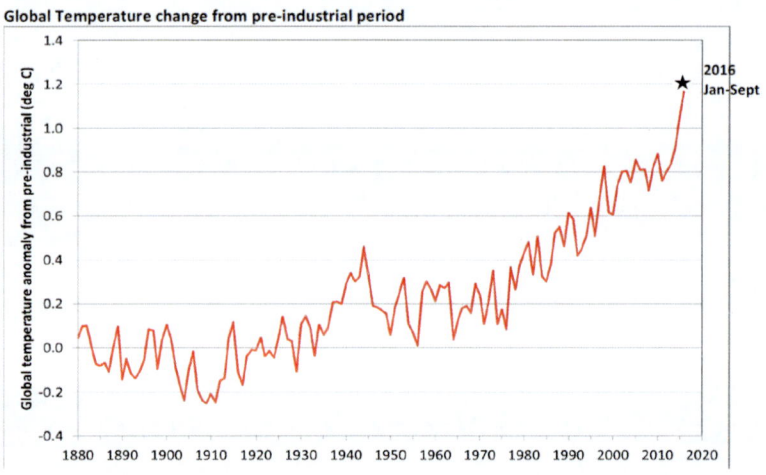

Figure 6.4: The rise in average global temperature from post-industrial revolution; 1880 to 2016.
[Figure adopted after permission obtained from concerned authorities] [11].

The culprit gases released by these unplanned industries into the atmosphere are called greenhouse gases. Moreover, the phenomenon by which they trap warmth in the atmosphere prevents it from escaping into space, resulting in global warming, called the "Greenhouse Effect." These gases are mentioned in Table 2.1 [13].

Table 6.2:. Greenhouse gases [13]

- Carbon Dioxide (CO_2),
- Methane (CH_4),
- Ozone (O_3),
- Water Vapor (H_2O),
- Nitrous Oxide (N_2O),
- Fluorinated gases: These include the following gases:
- Hydrofluorocarbons (HFCs),
- Perfluorocarbons (PFCs),
- Sulfur hexafluoride (SF_6),
- Nitrogen trifluoride (NF_3).

The greenhouse effect is a natural phenomenon that makes life on the planet viable. Natural warmth is necessary to prevent the planet from freezing. However, the "human enhanced greenhouse effect," which is resultantly known as global warming, is due to the swift and significantly increased emissions of these greenhouse gases from factories and motor vehicles, due to their combustion of the fossil fuels "coal, oil, and natural gas" as energy reserves, as well as other sources being aerosols, etc. The phenomenon by which the greenhouse gases warm the air and earth by trapping heat energy from the sun within the atmosphere is depicted in Figure 6.5 [14].

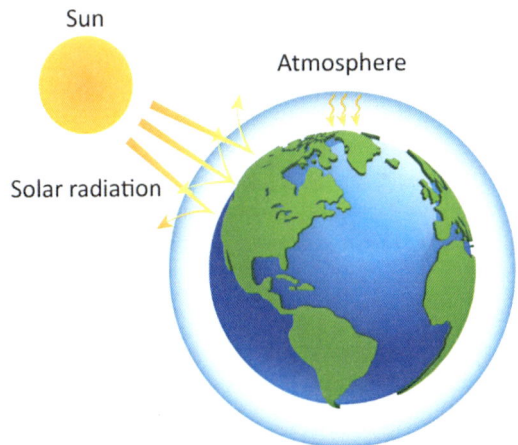

Figure 6.5: The phenomenon of the greenhouse effect.

There are different concentrations of greenhouse gases in the atmosphere, and the amount of heat each gas can trap varies greatly; this element is known as the Global Warming Potential. Figure 6.6 summarizes this information [15, 16]. The increased emissions of CO_2 since 1850, from different countries around the world, with the main source being the developed, or most populous, nations. This increase correlates with the rise of the global temperature depicted in Figure 6.4.

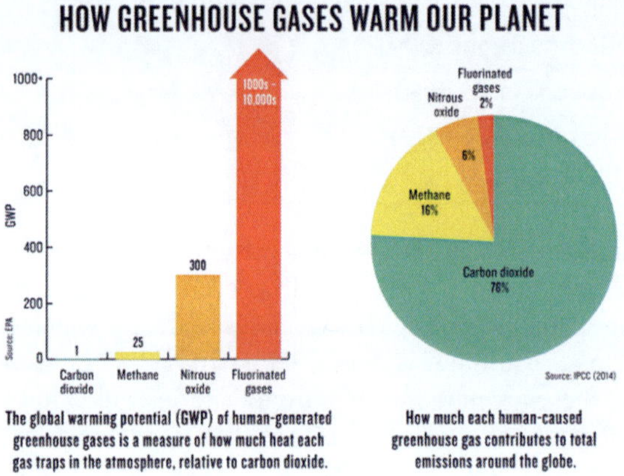

HOW GREENHOUSE GASES WARM OUR PLANET

The global warming potential (GWP) of human-generated greenhouse gases is a measure of how much heat each gas traps in the atmosphere, relative to carbon dioxide.

How much each human-caused greenhouse gas contributes to total emissions around the globe.

Figure 6.6: The power of contribution of each greenhouse gas to the greenhouse effect (GWP) vs. the emission of each greenhouse gas in the atmosphere from human activities [17].

Table 6.3 shows the rate of increased emissions of other greenhouse gases since preindustrial times: The concentrations of CO_2 (ppm), CH4 (parts per billion, ppb) and N2O (ppb), their growth rates (ppm/year for CO_2, ppb/year for CH4 and N2O) averaged over 2015–2017 and 2011–2015, the relative change in growth rates between 2011–2015 and 2015–2017, and the percentage of 2015–2017 concentration to preindustrial concentration (before 1750). Source: WMO Global Atmosphere Watch [17].

Table 6.3. Emissions of greenhouse gases

	Concentration			Growth rate		
	2015-2017	2011-2015	2015-2017 % to pre-industrial	2015-2017	2011-2015	% change
CO_2	403	395.5	145	2.6	2.2	+18%
CH_4	1851.7	1826.4	256	8.7	7.2	+21%
N_2O	329.1	326.2	122	0.87	0.73	+19%

Given the detailed statistics above, mathematical equations [18] reveal how the total greenhouse gas emissions per year (**T**) are dependent on the product presented in Table 6. 4.

Table 6.4. Mathematical equation to calculate greenhouse gas emissions per year [18].

- **P** = Population
- **C** = Consumption
- **E** = Greenhouse gas emissions per service

  T = P x C x E

With such a paradigm, where the global population is soaring uncontrollably, and so is the consumption per human being. The greenhouse emissions have been tried to put under control by limiting the E of the equation, that is, the emissions per service. This has been done by introducing zero-emission energy technologies such as renewables and advanced nuclear energy [19]. With some disadvantages compared to the non-renewable energy sources of coal, oil, and natural gas, which have been the main culprits of global warming for centuries now, this is perhaps the best solution humans have to prevent further damage to their planet's environment. Thus, life on this planet is damaged significantly. However, given the increasing demands for a better living by the modern world, these prospects seem hard to meet, and no nation is ready to make the sacrifice.

Various elements of nature and the ecosystem are being disturbed by global warming. They will continue to do so in the future at accelerated rates, given the pace of global development. As high above as the ozone layer of our planet's environment is being affected, mainly due to gases such as CFCs. With significant planning but limited application, there seems to be little human intervention to stop the damage to our world. Perhaps this is why nature had to intervene, to protect itself, by putting a halt to human activities. Hence, just when the advanced 21st century world seemed well equipped for any calamity, along came a God-sent intervention: COVID-19. A pandemic due to a minuscule, invisible to the naked eye, virus brought the entire global population of 7.7 billion to a halt. This pandemic undoubtedly had a disastrous impact on the life of every single human being, but perhaps the only good it brought along was of that to the climate and global environment. The impact of COVID-19 on climate change will be discussed in the next section.

Impact of the Pandemic on Climate Change and Global Warming

Ever since the world went into a global lockdown in 2020, after the spread of the COVID-19 pandemic, morbidity, mortality, the collapse of giant economies, suspension of travel, and closure of international borders, was experienced by all, thereby restricting every person to the walls of their own homes, while witnessing the chaos in the world outside through their T.V. screens. Adopting rules and regulations for health safety, witnessing the cessation of everyday life, social distancing, and isolating upon the slightest of flu symptoms that, previously, had held no significance, the COVID-19 pandemic weighed most upon its victims and especially the health care system and its workers.

While every single person struggled to adapt to the changing world as the "new normal," the heaviest price had to be paid by doctors, nurses, and medical staff, who over the past year, to date, have been fighting on the frontlines, isolated from their families and waging war against the virus while forsaking their lives to treat the patients of COVID-19. Given the duty of working in an exposed environment, not only were these frontliners in months of separation from their loved ones, but a significant number of health care workers around the world lost their lives to this pandemic while saving the lives of others.

Clean air, unpolluted blue skies, a greener environment, and crystal-clear water bodies resulted. Whereas human beings suffered and grieved the loss of life, the planet and nature, on the other hand, experienced an opposite reform. It was the first time people in India could see the Himalayas for the first time in "decades," as the lockdown eased air pollution, a report on CNN stated [20].

Given the months of global lockdown and the highest cases of COVID-19 in the most developed countries of the world, such as China, the United States, and the United Kingdom, these very nations with perhaps the highest rate of development and industrialization, were forced to shut down completely. The nations which have been the top 10 emitters of greenhouse gases are China, the USA, the European Union, India, the Russian Federation, Indonesia, Brazil, Japan, Canada, and Mexico [21].

Since workplaces, schools, universities, and all forms of social life were shut down, crowded roads and transport vehicles became a sight rare to see. This lockdown, that forcefully brought a halt to all human activities, significantly impacted the environment. Above all, factories and industries were sealed for a long period, thereby drastically reducing the emissions of CO_2 and other greenhouse gases from the factories into the atmosphere. Even though this short-lived decrease in CO_2 emissions was likely to have no significant consequences for global warming and climate change, in the long run, the decline, if maintained, could lead the planet onto the road to recovery from damage that started centuries ago.

It is not that the world has never seen death in such large numbers before. Previous pandemics [22], such as the HIV/AIDS pandemic between 2005 and 2012, resulted in a death toll of 36 million, and the Asian Flu pandemic in 1968 lead to approximately 1 million deaths. However, it can be said that such a mass lockdown is being seen for the first time in history since, given the degree of globalization, where traveling from one end of the world to the other is simply a matter of a few hours, the world over the past decade has become more connected than ever. Given the easy transfer of the virus and the disease, it became compulsory that strict shutdown policies had to be implemented immediately across cities, across international borders, and in the air space.

Considering this, it is not true that a decline in CO_2 emissions has been unprecedented. However, no world war, no crisis, and no previous pandemic has ever brought such a dramatic decline before. This indicates the weight and impact of COVID-19 itself. Dr. Glen Peters, research director at the Centre for International Climate Research (CICERO) in Norway, told a press briefing: "You would have to go back to 1945, the second world war, to see a relative drop bigger than this 7%." This year has also seen the first apparent fall in global emissions since a 1.3% drop in 2009, which was driven by the global financial crisis that started in 2008 [23, 24]. The literature shows that the emissions of CO_2, greenhouse gases over the years and how the graph suddenly falls in 2020 owing to the pandemic shutdown.

The CO_2 emissions for the initial months of 2020 more closely, when the pandemic first spread worldwide. Given the decline experienced this year, the decline in greenhouse gas emissions, if maintained for 10 more years till 2030, can reverse the 1.5-2°C rise in average global temperature that is termed as "global warming."

This fall in emissions is now termed as the "green recovery." Intense action can change this temperature trajectory. According to a report by the United Nations, the green recovery could cut expected emissions in 2030 by up to 25 percent and boost the chance of keeping temperature rise to below 2°C, up to 66 percent, according to the report [26]. However, the U.N. also states that despite the minute decline in global CO_2 emissions due to the pandemic, the planet will, however, be headed for a global temperature rise of over 3°C this century, due to the continuing emissions. The CO_2 emissions were declining in 2020 during the COVID-19 pandemic, and greenhouse emissions over the year were reduced, owing to COVID-19 and the estimated period to reverse the rise of global temperature of 1.5-2°C. The literature also proves how the pandemic considerably slowed down the release of greenhouse gases in the atmosphere, such as a study published in Nature Communications, conducted at the beginning of 2020, by Liu et al. [27] titled "Near-real-time monitoring of global CO_2 emissions reveals the effects of the COVID-19 pandemic." This research analyzed region-specific estimates of daily CO_2 emissions that were measured from hourly data collection from electric power production, daily vehicle traffic, daily international passenger flights and distance flown, monthly production data for industrial output, and fuel consumption data combined with weather information for residential and commercial building emissions and then interpreted the substantial COVID-related decreases in CO_2 emissions between January 1 and June 30 of 2020 as compared to 2019. In the aggregate, emissions were 8.8% lower, where the daily CO_2 emissions time series revealed that the different timings of the reductions were synchronous with lockdown measures. They also showed how in the first half of 2020, the most pronounced decline occurred in the U.S (−13.3%), followed by EU27 & U.K. (−12.7%), India (−15.4%), and China (−3.7%), with substantial but progressive decreases in Japan (−7.5%), Russia (−5.3%) and Brazil (−12.0%). The sudden, large, and early drop of Chinese emissions corresponds to the initial outbreak of COVID-19 and the country's strict lockdown measures, which were gradually relaxed in March 2020, and again lockdown measures were implemented during the second wave in December 2020.

Simultaneously, the study also revealed the lack of acknowledgment and appreciation by nations worldwide for this improvement in the health of the planet due to the pandemic, since soon after the cases dropped in certain countries, not only did their CO_2 emission surge once again but also crossed the peak of the previous year. The same study by Liu et al. 2020 [27] shows how China's CO_2 emissions soon recovered quickly, where monthly relative differences between 2020-2019 were −18.4% in February, −9.2% in March, +0.6% (i.e., greater in 2020 than 2019) in April, and reached +5.4% in May, indicating a rebound above 2019 in the same month of the year [28].

There have been multiple agreements worldwide made on big international forums to bring a slow down to the process of climate change, such as the Paris Agreement that is a legally binding international treaty on climate change. This was adopted by 196 parties in Paris on December 12, 2015, and entered into force on November 4, 2016, with its goal being "to limit global warming to well below 2, preferably to 1.5 degrees Celsius, compared to preindustrial levels" [29].

However, evidence of such data reveals how despite the urgency of the situation and the tremendous amount of awareness that is being raised regarding global warming, nations around the globe are not applying these policies strictly and perhaps are not ready to make the sacrifices required to heal the damage caused by human beings themselves. The cause to reverse the effects of climate change requires joint efforts by all countries, especially developed nations, around the world, to switch to more expensive but renewable energy sources, reduce the amount of non-renewable fuel used, spread further awareness about the existence and adverse effects of climate change, global warming and air/water pollution to citizens via mass media campaigns, and avoid activities such as deforestation, that lead to further damage to the ecosystem. Such interventions will come at the cost of certain sacrifices that may affect the rate of development, especially of the competing developed nations, due to the focus being shifted to bettering, not their economies, but the planet. However, perhaps human beings must intercede to stop this damage and learn from the positive outcomes from a calamity such as COVID-19, before we have other disasters sent our way that damage human life, and the planet, irreparably.

After all, Planet Earth is our only home.

Reversing roles: Impact of the climate on the pandemic itself. Is there any? We have discussed the various influences the pandemic has had and how it continues to impact on different spheres of life on this planet, including the climate. However, the question also arises, what if we reverse roles and investigate the impact that the environment itself has had on the COVID-19 situation worldwide. Have countries with different temperatures and weather patterns experienced morbidity and mortality rates due to a lack of implementation of strict policies by the public, or has there been any variation in the slightest, due to the climate and temperature itself on these numbers?

While there were rumors that COVID-19 rates would drop worldwide in the summer of 2020 due to heat destroying the virus, while the cases would spike once again in winter, due to the cold and higher incidences of other infections common in winter, such as the common cold and pneumonia, evidence is now building up that there has been some truth to these rumors.

A study conducted by Wu et al. 2020 [30] in the United States showed that people living in poorer air conditions had higher fatality rates with COVID-19. They found an increase of only 1 $\mu g/m^3$ in PM2.5 was associated with an 8% increase in the COVID-19 death rate (95% confidence interval [CI]: 2%, 15%). Given the fact that poorer air quality leads to a higher chance, and incidence of, respiratory infections, it is only natural that the following results were proven.

Another study, conducted in China by Tang et al., [31] shows the same result, that poorer air quality in China may have increased transmission of infections that cause influenza-like illnesses. Another study by Zhao et al. [32] found that multiple viruses, including the adenovirus and influenza viruses, can be transmitted and carried on air particles showing particulate matter that likely contributed to the spread of the 2015 avian influenza.

The studies above mentioned the impact air pollution has on the pandemic and its numbers. Certain studies also targeted how different temperatures and humidity levels in different states have led to fluctuations in those areas. A study conducted by Meo et al. 2020 [33] shows how heat and humidity affected COVID-19 in the ten biggest European countries. The authors concluded that an increase in relative humidity was linked to a decrease in the number of daily cases and deaths. However, a temperature rise was allied with an upsurge in the number of daily cases and daily deaths due to the COVID-19 pandemic. In Table 6.2, data obtained from this study shows the effect of temperature and humidity on the number of daily cases and fatalities, and cumulative cases and deaths due to COVID-19, in these 10 European countries.

Table 6.5: Temperature, humidity, number of daily cases, cumulative cases, daily deaths, and cumulative deaths due to the COVID-19 pandemic in European countries (permission obtained from both author and publisher to reuse this table).

Countries	Temperature °C (mean ± SEM)	Humidity % (mean ± SEM)	Daily Cases (mean ± SEM)	Cumulative Cases (mean ± SEM)	Daily Deaths (mean ± SEM)	Cumulative Deaths (mean ± SEM)
Russia	11.58 ± 0.73	59.79 ± 1.55	4492.33 ± 316.73	221994.73 ± 20133.13	71.73 ± 5.61	2910.13 ± 292.70
United Kingdom	16.56 ± 0.44	55.97 ± 1.41	1737.31 ± 239.34	141853.67 ± 9701.21	266.97 ± 32.60	20242.77 ± 1421.50
Spain	22.73 ± 0.59	47.32 ± 1.52	1535.30 ± 172.25	144515.35 ± 8162.83	195.56 ± 23.80	16076.84 ± 947.54
Italy	21.69 ± 0.46	50.35 ± 1.17	1425.35 ± 134.00	140949.22 ± 7634.66	204.77 ± 19.11	19454.39 ± 1114.02
Germany	15.77 ± 0.50	52.94 ± 1.49	1167.69 ± 125.26	107958.17 ± 6239.47	52.80 ± 5.89	4435.39 ± 298.82
Turkey	20.85 ± 0.59	46.08 ± 1.55	1668.25 ± 107.41	120192.20 ± 6380.17	41.84 ± 3.14	3151.66 ± 171.75
France	16.56 ± 0.43	58.57 ± 1.32	938.80 ± 103.17	84509.58 ± 5039.22	170.63 ± 22.95	15398.05 ± 995.18
Belgium	15.84 ± 0.44	57.18 ± 1.43	381.13 ± 38.99	33812.28 ± 2032.35	59.02 ± 7.56	5190.72 ± 336.21
Netherlands	16.07 ± 0.42	59.45 ± 1.33	361.23 ± 31.78	32203.95 ± 1590.58	43.15 ± 4.61	3892.99 ± 206.07
Belarus	13.00 ± 0.63	59.59 ± 1.66	465.41 ± 40.48	26236.71 ± 2102.62	3.44 ± 0.24	161.52 ± 13.27
Mean ± SEM	17.07 ± 0.18	54.78 ± 0.47	14445.61 ± 59.34	107814.61 ± 3192.75	116.09 ± 5.87	9520.72 ± 309.06

Data presented from the date of appearance of first case of SARS-COV-2 in European countries, Jan 27, 2020 to July 17, 2020 Values are presented in Mean and SEM. Temperature °C: Humidity %.

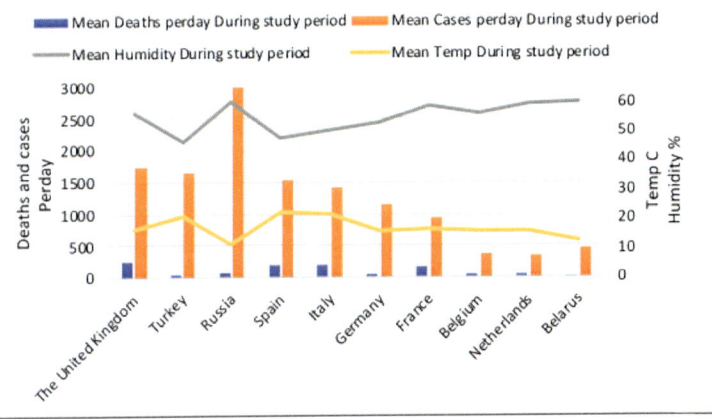

Figure 6.7: Mean temperature, humidity, number of daily cases, and daily deaths due to the COVID-19 pandemic in European countries. [Figure adopted after permission obtained from author and publisher] [33].

In another series of eye-opening research, it has also been marvelously shown how the wildfire in California, a devastating after-effect of human-induced global warming itself, led to increased mortality rates of patients with COVID-19 due to the smoke and particulate matter the wildfire created in those states. This study conducted by Meo et al. 2020 [34] reported that due to the wildfire in 10 different counties of California, PM2.5 concentration increased by 220.71%; O_3 by 19.56%; and the C.O. concentration increased by 151.05%. After the wildfire, the number of cases and deaths due to COVID-19 increased by 56.9% and 148.2%. Therefore, the California wildfire caused an increase in ambient concentrations of toxic pollutants, which were associated with an increase in the incidence and mortality rates of COVID-19.

Such studies and literature highlight the massive impact that our environment and surroundings have on our well-being. With this pandemic, we have closely seen the association of the environment on our health and, in reverse, the impact of human activities on the environment and wildlife. What have we done to our planet in the vicious cycle of bettering lives? Did we forget how the process was linked to the proportional damage to our ecosystem? The hopes have not died out yet. The possible solutions to what we can do to head to the road of betterment are discussed in the next section.

The Road to Betterment

The world of the 21st century is highly developed. With new technological advancements, there have been innovations and discoveries that man could never possibly think of even thinking. Then how could a little virus bring the world to a complete halt? Why did no one see this coming? Why were we not prepared for such a pandemic beforehand? These are questions that the world and scientific community must address. Nevertheless, so far, how do we prevent the pandemic and climate allied condition that has long set in and has been slowly eating away at our planet – global warming?

As mentioned continuously throughout this chapter, countries must take steps to possibly slow down, if not completely stop, the process of climate change that's gradually accelerating with time.

1. We can start with the most significant issue: greenhouse gas emissions. These must be reduced to the supreme if we are to head towards the road to recovery. We can make this possible by decreasing the consumption per individual, or by slowing down the global population's growth. Fewer greenhouse gases means less trapping of heat in the earth, thus slowing the process of temperature rise!

2. Switching to renewable energy sources instead of relying on the non-renewable fuels, coal, oil, and natural gas is, by far, one of the best ways to reduce CO_2 emissions, for these fuels are the primary source of greenhouse gases, via their combustion. This method involves solar power, wind turbines, geothermal energy, tidal energy, and nuclear energy, all of which can be utilized, as suited to each country and its available resources. By this means, we can be headed towards a green recovery by using "low carbon energy."

3. Management of refrigeration usage for they are the main source of ozone depletion caused by the CFCs they release.

4. Projects of reforestation of planting more trees worldwide shall preserve our environment and provide the habitats lost to animals by deforestation. This shall, in turn, prevent the extinction of species and the loss of biodiversity.

5. The establishment of international organizations and treaties, such as those under the United Nations and World Meteorological Organization or the United Nations Environment Programme, to construct standard models to ensure how GHG emissions' global levels, mainly CO_2, can be reduced. This may involve setting limits for countries to prevent them from exceeding the peak level of emissions and placing trade embargos, or restrictions, on them if they fail to comply with the implemented policies.

6. Creation of investigation committees that monitor the levels of CO_2 emitted globally, and per country.

7. Mass education of the global population, especially females, in order to educate future generations about the do's and don'ts they must apply to their lives to prevent the harm their ancestors caused to the planet is pivotal to changing an individual's perspective to everything.

8. Mass media and social media campaigns to spread awareness about climate change, its impact on us, its adverse effects, and what we can do to prevent it.

9. Providing habitats to endangered species around the globe and taking measures to ensure they do not become extinct.

10. Reconstruction of our agricultural practices to ensure that the population's sufficient dietary demands are met without posing a threat or damaging the environment.

11. Preserving water, via the construction of dams and reservoirs, in the periods of heavy spells of rainfall and educating the public to conserve water to avoid a crisis in the future.

12. Emphasis on preventing the human-based pollution of land and water bodies.

13. Preventing unwanted toxic materials from being dispersed into the atmosphere, whether air or water, by making safe disposal sites for waste. Avoiding air pollution (via nitrogen oxides, sulfur dioxide, and carbon dioxide), which has been shown to lead to an increased incidence of heart attacks, strokes as well as obesity, diabetes, and premature deaths that put further strains on our economies and health care systems.

14. Funding of governments into research for creating strategies to pave the road to the green recovery and better human living and life on the planet, simultaneously.

Conclusion

In summary, besides the solutions mentioned above, we must learn from, and implement, the lessons taught to us by the COVID-19 pandemic. We must ask ourselves the questions of how we lacked, where we lacked, and what steps we can take to avoid such a calamity and so much loss of life in the future. Millions have grieved the loss of loved ones, and the new decade's dawn brought a change to the world never witnessed before. We have watched how helpless humanity is in front of the Divine Decree. Hence, if society cannot think, reflect and take heed from so much suffering over the past year, then perhaps nothing can change us. For the will comes from within us. Maybe together, however, step by step, we can have hope that someday our targets can be met, and our dreams can be achieved. Thus, maybe shortly, we can hope that we will head towards recovery. That life on this planet can go back to being as peaceful as our ancestors' once was.

References

1. Who.int. 2021. Archived: WHO Timeline - COVID-19. [online] Available at: <https://www.who.int/news/item/27-04-2020-who-timeline---covid-19> [Accessed 8 January 2021].

2. Worldometers.info. 2021. Coronavirus Update (Live): 94,775,478 Cases And 2,027,067 Deaths From COVID-19 Virus Pandemic - Worldometer. [online] Available at: <https://www.worldometers.info/coronavirus/> [Accessed 8 January 2021].

3. Pfizer.com. 2021. Coronavirus Disease (COVID-19) Facts, News & Information | Pfizer. [online] Available at: <https://www.pfizer.com/health/coronavirus> [Accessed 8 January 2021].

4. The Guardian. 2021. Covid Cases Recorded In Antarctica For First Time – Reports. [online] Available at: <https://www.theguardian.com/world/2020/dec/22/covid-cases-recorded-in-antarctica-for-first-time> [Accessed 16 January 2021].

5. Worldometers.info. 2021. Coronavirus Update (Live): 94,794,002 Cases And 2,027,629 Deaths From COVID-19 Virus Pandemic - Worldometer. [online] Available at: <https://www.worldometers.info/coronavirus/> [Accessed 8 January 2021].

6. En.wikipedia.org. 2021. History Of Climate Change Science. [online] Available at: <https://en.wikipedia.org/wiki/History_of_climate_change_science> [Accessed 16 January 2021].

7. Climate-science.com. 2021. Climate Change Is Bad. How Bad?. [online] Available at: <https://climate-science.com/advanced-crash-course-climate-change/> [Accessed 16 January 2021].

8. Library.wmo.int. 2021. [online] Available at: <https://library.wmo.int/doc_num.php?explnum_id=9936> [Accessed 16 January 2021].

9. Future_We_Don't_Want_Report_1.4_hi-res_120618.original.pdf C40-production-images.s3.amazonaws.com. 2021. [online] Available at: <https://c40-production-images.s3.amazonaws.com/other_uploads/images/1789_Future_We_Don't_Want_Report_1.4_hi-res_120618.original.pdf> [Accessed 16 January 2021].

10. The Guardian. 2021. How Will Climate Change Affect Rainfall? [online] Available at <https://www.theguardian.com/environment/2011/dec/15/climate-change-rainfall> [Accessed January 16th, 2021].

11. World Meteorological Organization. 2021. COP22 Advances Global Action On Climate Change. [online] Available at: https://public.wmo.int/en/resources/meteoworld/cop22-advances-global-action-climate-change [Accessed 16 January 2021].

12. Alan Buis, &., 2021. Milankovitch (Orbital) Cycles And Their Role In Earth's Climate – Climate Change: Vital Signs Of The Planet. [online] Climate Change: Vital Signs of the Planet. Available at: <https://climate.nasa.gov/news/2948/milankovitch-orbital-cycles-and-their-role-in-earths-climate/> [Accessed 16 January 2021].

13. NRDC. 2021. Greenhouse Effect 101. [online] Available at: <https://www.nrdc.org/stories/greenhouse-effect-101> [Accessed 16 January 2021].

14. ThurstonTalk. 2021. Home Science Activities With South Sound GREEN: Climate Controllers - Thurstontalk. [online] Available at: <https://www.thurstontalk.com/2020/07/16/home-science-activities-with-south-sound-green-climate-controllers/> [Accessed 16 January 2021].

15. NRDC. 2021. Greenhouse Effect 101. [online] Available at: <https://www.nrdc.org/stories/greenhouse-effect-101> [Accessed 16 January 2021].

16. Nytimes.com. 2021. Teach About Climate Change With These 24 New York Times Graphs (Published 2019). [online] Available at: <https://www.nytimes.com/2019/02/28/learning/teach-about-climate-change-

with-these-24-new-york-times-graphs.html> [Accessed 16 January 2021].

17. 2021. The Global Climate in 2015–2019. [ebook] Geneva: Chairperson, Publications Board, p.4. Available at: <https://library.wmo.int/doc_num.php?explnum_id=9936> [Accessed 2 January 2021].

18. IPCC, 2014: Summary for Policymakers. In: Climate Change 2014: Mitigation of Climate Change. Contribution of Working Group III to the Fifth Assessment Report of the Intergovernmental Panel on Climate Change [Edenhofer, O., R. Pichs-Madruga, Y. Sokona, E. Farahani, S. Kadner, K. Seyboth, A. Adler, I. Baum, S. Brunner, P. Eickemeier, B. Kriemann, J. Savolainen, S. Schlömer, C. von Stechow, T. Zwickel and J.C. Minx (eds.)]. Cambridge University Press, Cambridge, United Kingdom and New York, NY, USA.

19. Hannah Ritchie and Max Roser (2017) – "CO_2 and Greenhouse Gas Emissions". Published online at OurWorldInData.org. Retrieved from: "https://ourworldindata.org/co2-and-other-greenhouse-gas-emissions" [Online Resource]

20. Rob Picheta, C., 2021. People in India can see the Himalayas for the first time in 'decades,' as the lockdown eases air pollution. [online] CNN. Available at: <https://www.cnn.com/travel/article/himalayas-visible-lockdown-india-scli-intl/index.html> [Accessed January 3rd 2021].

21. World Resources Institute. 2021. CAIT: WRI's climate data explorer. [online] Available at: <https://cait.wri.org/historical/Country%20GHG%20Emissions> [Accessed 6 January 2021].

22. Mphonline.org. 2021. Outbreak: 10 of the Worst Pandemics in History. [online] Available at: <https://www.mphonline.org/worst-pandemics-in-history/> [Accessed 7 January 2021].

23. Carbon Brief. 2021. Global Carbon Project: Coronavirus causes record fall in fossil-fuel emissions in 2020 | Carbon Brief. [online] Available at: <https://www.carbonbrief.org/global-carbon-project-coronavirus-causes-record-fall-in-fossil-fuel-emissions-in-2020> [Accessed 7 January 2021].

24. Earth.Org - Past | Present | Future. 2021. 'Extreme' 17% Drop in Global Carbon Emissions Due to COVID-19 Shutdowns | Earth.Org - Past | Present | Future. [online] Available at: <https://earth.org/covid-19-drop-carbon-emissions/> [Accessed 9 January 2021].

25. Unctad.org. 2021. COVID-19 stalls progress on Global Goals | UNCTAD. [online] Available at: <https://unctad.org/es/node/3067> [Accessed 8 January 2021].

26. U.N. News. 2021. 'Green recovery' from COVID-19 can slow climate change: U.N. environment report. [online] Available at: <https://news.un.org/en/story/2020/12/1079602> [Accessed 19 January 2021].

27. Liu, Z., Ciais, P., Deng, Z. et al. Near-real-time monitoring of global CO_2 emissions reveals the effects of the COVID-19 pandemic. Nat Commun 2020; 5172. https://doi.org/10.1038/s41467-020-18922-7.

28. Carbon Brief. 2021. Analysis: China's CO_2 emissions surged past pre-coronavirus levels in May. [online] Available at: <https://www.carbonbrief.org/analysis-chinas-co2-emissions-surged-past-pre-coronavirus-levels-in-may> [Accessed 9 January 2021].

29. Unfccc.int. 2021. [online] Available at: <https://unfccc.int/process-and-meetings/the-paris-agreement/the-paris-agreement> [Accessed 11 January 2021].

30. Wu X, Nethery RC, Sabbath BM, Braun D, Dominici F. Exposure to air pollution and COVID-19 mortality in the United States: A nationwide cross-sectional study. Preprint. medRxiv. 2020;2020.04.05.20054502. doi:10.1101/2020.04.05.20054502

31. Tang S, Yan Q, Shi W, Wang X, Sun X, Yu P, Wu J, Xiao Y. Measuring the impact of air pollution on respiratory infection risk in China. Environmental Pollution, 2018; 232: 477-486.

32. Zhao Y, Richardson B, Takl, E, Chai L, Schmitt D, Xin H. Airborne transmission may have played a role in spreading 2015 highly pathogenic avian influenza outbreaks in the United States. Scientific Reports, 2019; 9: 11755. https://doi.org/10.1038/s41598-019-47788-z.

33. Meo SA, Abukhalaf AA, Alomar AA, Sumaya OY, Sami W, Shafi KM, Meo AS, Usmani AM, Akram J. Effect of heat and humidity on the incidence and mortality due to COVID-19 pandemic in European countries. Eur Rev Med Pharmacol Sci. 2020; 24 (17): 9216-9225. doi: 10.26355/eurrev_202009_22874. PMID: 32965017.

34. Meo S, Abukhalaf A, Alomar A, Alessa O, Sami W, Klonoff D. Effect of environmental pollutants PM-2.5, carbon monoxide, and ozone on the incidence and mortality of SARS-COV-2 infection in ten wildfire affected counties in California. Science of The Total Environment, 2021; 757: 143948.

COVID-19 Pandemic: Challenges to Frontline Health Care Workers

Nadia Naseem

Abstract

The novel coronavirus SARS-CoV-2 infection, originating from the Hubei Province of the People's Republic of China, was reported as a worldwide health emergency; the World Health Organization (WHO) declared the SARS-CoV-2 infection as a global pandemic (COVID-19). In a short time, SARS-CoV-2 spread across the entire world. However, frontline health care workers, including medical, para-medical, and laboratory staff, face great difficulties while performing their duties. This chapter explores the challenges faced by the frontline health care workers during the COVID-19 pandemic.

Keywords: COVID-19, Frontline Workers, Health Care Workers, Global Challenges.

Introduction

In the context of the global crisis caused by the COVID-19 pandemic, health care workers are the first line of defense to combat this pandemic. They face this health emergency with poor working conditions, lack of adequate resources, shortage of biosafety equipment, inadequate infection control systems, lack of recognition programs and work incentives, physical and psychological abuse, and discrimination by the patients, which have negative implications on their mental health also. Unquestionably, the pandemic did not influence all countries likewise; the ones to suffer most were those with a split health system, financial debts, considerable geographic and population strength, and socio-cultural issues related to access to health care services, deficits in infrastructure, a dearth of equipment and trained human resources in hospitals [1]. With the ongoing spread of the pandemic, many intensive care health workers shifted to new jobs leaving the critical care centers in the hands of young volunteers who were less trained, and unfamiliar with the realistic demands of the ICUs and emergency duties. The burden of training and supervising these volunteers fell on already stressed senior clinicians who had to work in the critical care centers for long hours, thus, frequently acquiring COVID-19 infection. The world lost many of its revered and highly skilled consultants during this pandemic. The role of laboratories increased manifold during the pandemic, with subsequent heavy workloads and turnover of RT-PCR testing throughout the world. This diversion of practice led to a sheer compromise in the turnaround time of routine tests because of the heavy commitment of staff towards the emergency reporting of SARS-CoV-2 results. Moreover, most routine laboratories upgraded to BSL-2/3 level laboratories to handle the common specimens and gain lucrative benefits from SARS-CoV-2 testing.

The worldwide decline in life expectancy, from continuing exposure to ambient air pollution, surpasses that of infectious diseases compared to that of tobacco smoking. The mortality from COVID-19 depends mainly on comorbidities, including arterial hypertension, diabetes mellitus, obesity, coronary artery disease, and respiratory conditions such as asthma and chronic obstructive pulmonary disease (COPD) [2]. Continued exposure to air pollution has been associated with acute respiratory inflammation, asthma attack, and death from cardiopulmonary diseases in the past literature. Fine particulate matter (particles with aerodynamic diameters less than 2.5 μm, PM2.5) is considered one of the foremost environmental health risk factors, causing millions of casualties per year globally [3]. Particulate matter increases the activity of the ACE-2 receptor, thus causing a '*double hit*' mechanism: air pollution causes the destruction of lungs and increases the activity of ACE-2, thus causing an increase in uptake of the virus by the lungs, blood vessels, and the heart [4]. Several studies [5-7] indicate a negative correlation of COVID 19 with specific environmental parameters, including temperature, humidity, precipitation, and wind speed; however, a positive relation was seen with air quality. The significance of air quality suggests that green environment strategies should be encouraged to limit the transmission of infectious diseases like COVID-19.

Even though confounding factors could be present (for example, age of exposed individuals, gender, and smoking), the probability of a harmful effect of air pollution on the prognosis of patients affected by COVID-19 is likely, and merits further investigation. Therefore, a global effort is necessary in terms of the organization of collaborative networks and the implementation of universal emergency strategies.

The world is in a state of war against the pandemic of SARS-CoV-2, and casualties are increasing drastically across the globe, resulting in international travel restrictions, the withdrawal of significant sporting occasions, and the lockdown of borders having a major influence on the global economy. This crisis is expected to have longer-term economic effects. Unemployment has increased the risk that many people will become stuck in unemployment, particularly affecting younger workers and lower-skilled workers. The closure of schools and universities has created education crises. Moreover, the stock exchange and crude oil rates have dropped markedly. Industries associated with entertainment, ceremonial events, hotels, and tourism are also influenced. The lockdown, and other related limitations, have rigorously affected the economic status and the welfare of families and communities. In short, the chief sectors targeted by this pandemic are health, education, manufacturing, transportation, and trade, among many others [8]. Public health strategies adopted against this pandemic have created alarming domestic violence and mental health issues [9].

A novel coronavirus infection, named COVID-19, was first spotted in Wuhan city, China, in December 2019, becoming a global public health issue due to its rapid spread. It was reported as a pandemic by the World Health Organization in March 2020[10]. The ongoing changes in climate, particularly global warming, and the recent damage caused by the coronavirus have been controversial virtually worldwide. Past studies have concluded that air pollution is a significant risk factor for respiratory tract infections by transmitting microorganisms, thus worsening the body's immunity. It has been reported that people who live in areas with poor air quality are expected to die more from COVID-19, even when considering other factors that may affect the possibility of death, such as pre-existing medical conditions, socioeconomic status, and approach to health care facilities[11]. Similar results were obtained in other studies, which concluded that a slight increase in the exposure to PM2.5 results in a massive rise in COVID-19 mortality rates [12, 13].

COVID-19 Pandemic and Frontline Health Care Workers

Globally, the frontline health care workers were the most affected professionals among the rest of the occupational workers. The work-life of the doctors, paramedics, and janitorial staff working in hospital settings has changed vividly with increasing demand for physical, mental, social, and financial challenges imposed by the pandemic, and its sequel. This was besides struggling to counter the fear of contagion and keeping their loved ones and family at home safe. Immense social and emotional pressure from families and friends to quit their jobs led to alarming negative physical and mental implications on these frontline workers. The discomfort was borne further by continuously wearing the personal protective equipment (PPE), including cover-suits, gloves, face masks and shields, earplugs, goggles, etc., according to their job and specialty requirements.

Furthermore, uninterrupted duty hours, the unpredictable outcome of the patients under their management, the sufferings of a large number of terminally ill patients left alone in ICUs, the colossal death toll, and dealing with the relatives of the dead, or dying, patients from diverse socio-cultural backgrounds, are curtailing their potential to work effectively, with rapid burnout [14, 15]. As reported by the World Health Organization, approximately 70% of the global health care workforce is comprised of women [16], of whom many had to face additional domestic and caregiving issues to maintain their work-life balance at an optimum. Numerous studies throughout the world reported emotional and psychological pressures and morbidities, including severe depression [17, 18], and suicidal tendencies among the doctors [19].

The doctors working as intensivists with the core skills of emergency and critical care medicine for managing ventilators, continuous renal replacement therapy (CRRT), ECMO (extracorporeal membrane oxygenation), ultrasound assessment, and tracheostomy suffered most from the pressures of job timing and infectivity during the pandemic [20]. Unfortunately, even the developed world faced a shortage of a continuous and adequate supply of beds, medicines, critical medical equipment, and PPEs for the health care workers. During the peak pandemic era, most of the time, the health care workers were buying the PPEs from their own pockets, or through the help of certain NGOs, to protect themselves while working with COVID-19 patients. Lack of funds and financial cut-backs in the budget allocated for the health care quota throughout the world resulted in a massive downsizing of health care workers. It increased workforce shortage in hospitals and other healthcare facilities, especially in rural areas [21].

A halt to educational and training activities led to the disruption of the academic progress of most of the trainees and residents, loss of tuition fees, missed exams, and potentially delayed certification, with the subsequent loss of opportunities for promotion and better jobs [22].

As stated by Benjamin Franklin *"By failing to prepare, you are preparing to fail"*; across the globe, the COVID-19 pandemic has made us learn a big lesson: that the preparedness of the institutions, and the devising of a crisis plan for timely action in case of unforeseen disasters or pandemics, is the key to the attainment of subsistence and survival. The whole world faced challenges related to the sustainability of the delivery of health services that gravely affected health care providers such as doctors, nurses, and allied health professionals [23, 24]. With time, all pro-active countries and governments planned flexible scheduling, teleworking through telemedicine, backup/emergency staff recruitment, and vast use of print and electronic media for public awareness and psychological support for the people and health workers. A considerable number of webinars, digital seminars, and training were planned to disseminate essential knowledge and inculcation of skills in managing the pandemic and affected patients in terms of isolation, clinical treatment, decontamination, communication, triaging psychological support, and palliative care [25-28]. Continuing education to health care workers, their families, and the wider public can help minimize the stigma and discrimination associated with COVID-19. Psychosocial support must be provided as a mandatory and readily available facility at all levels to augment the physical and mental capabilities of the health care providers during this critical time.

COVID-19 and Medical Teaching Faculty Challenges

The coronavirus (COVID-19) pandemic has disturbed the economy and social life globally, with more than three billion people during the lockdown. The outcome of this current pandemic will be a long-term transformation in medical education and is likely to have long-lasting consequences on student learning. Academic management has been placed under tremendous pressure in the delivery, access, and assessment of courses. Universities and colleges worldwide have been closed, affecting millions of students worldwide, and online education has abruptly become an academic norm. Under these circumstances, educators and students may find this rapid transition to online instruction disturbing and unsatisfying. Many teaching institutes across the world adopted online education tools and training to facilitate students in continuing their courses, thus safeguarding their academic year. Lately, the technological developments within the last few years, far-reaching accessibility, and uninterrupted connectivity ensured feasible and affordable approaches to remote education with the subsequent dissemination and interchange of knowledge and learning throughout the globe.

Nevertheless, many developed countries have entrenched online and distant-learning degree programs and short courses in place, which may be in contrast to the developing world where even medical schools, especially of the public sector, lack such facilities for the students, thus posing a great challenge for e-learning in these countries [29]. Challenges faced, due to the pandemic included those associated with communication, student evaluation, technology tools usage, online skill, anxiety or stress related to the pandemic, time management, and technophobia, leading to real challenges for low- and middle-income countries. In developing countries, most medical colleges have outdated syllabi; most of the senior teachers employed in the medical schools face serious issues in executing online education because of a lack of prior experience and insufficient training to participate in the arduous task of online education teaching each day. Distant education has always been fancied as an optional mode of teaching and learning; therefore, in this emergency crisis of the COVID-19 pandemic, unpreparedness and inadequate IT training are considered the ultimate barriers to implementing digital / e-learning educational programs in the world. Also, most of the world's rural population faced internet affordability and connectivity issues due to engagement in course coverage for long hours and repeated interruptions during video streaming and attending video conferences for lectures [30, 31]. Female faculty, especially, have faced many problems during working from home while synchronously maintaining a work-life balance throughout this worldwide pandemic. In countries with a conservative society and strong religious ties, female members of the family have an added duty of dealing with their household and looking after their children as a primary duty, thus leading to an additional physical and mental pressure and anxiety for females working and teaching from home during the COVID-19 crisis [29].

Several policies have been suggested to improve the quality of online teaching and augmenting student commitment. Many free online courses are available for educationalists to grasp the dynamics of online education and generate engaging sessions for the students. Additionally, several technology-boosted assessment methods are also accessible, and the faculty should command these technologies. Institutes with well-established information technology and medical education departments, and experience of effectively dealing with e-learning before the COVID-19 pandemic, should share their expertise and deliver guidance to new e-learning. Moreover, further research is required to officially document the experiences and challenges being encountered by the students and faculties in this crisis. There is a need to introduce policies suitable for the local work environment and learn from the experience of other skilled people. Historically, pandemics have caused challenges; the first step is to identify and convert them into opportunities. The key option is to involve the medical students and faculty in converting the existing pandemic-imposed remote medical teaching into an evidence-based model [32,33].

COVID-19 and Challenges faced by Health Care Laboratories

Autopsies and examinations should be performed, ideally in certified Biosafety Level 3 (BSL-3), or higher. It is not possible to establish a perfect environment in a short time in, or near, an epicenter, but with appropriate modifications, isolated accommodations, or operating rooms equipped with adequate facilities the required protection standards can be met [34]. As the worldwide COVID-19 pandemic continues to grow, global health care services necessitate adopting the latest approaches and re-adapting to the challenges posed by this novel respiratory virus. The Anatomic Pathology laboratory, which deals with human biological specimens, must also be prepared to deal with these challenges and continue to offer high-standard services to all the patients, while guaranteeing that its administrative staff, technicians, trainees, and pathologists work in a safe environment [35]. Each histopathology laboratory must perform a risk assessment of the available facilities; in the first step reviewing the routinely performed procedures, hazard identification in the processes and procedures, determining the competency level of the staff, and evaluating chemicals are required. After addressing the mitigation strategies, professional training and refresher workshops are mandatory for maintenance. Regular inspection and sustentation of chemicals and types of equipment in the laboratory clinches the process [36].

SARS-CoV-2 is classified as a risk group 3 pathogen; therefore, provisional guidelines from the CDC propose that Biosafety Level 2 (BSL-2) laboratory practices should be adopted while dealing with a specimen that might have SARS-CoV-2, which includes pathologic analysis and processing of formalin-fixed or fresh tissues, an ancillary study of extracted nucleic acid formulations, electron microscopic analysis with glutaraldehyde-fixed grids, a frequent examination of bacterial and mycotic cultures, daily staining and microscopic examination of fixed smears, ultimate packaging of samples for transport, and inactivation of tissues such as the insertion of specimens in a nucleic acid extraction buffer. In case of virus isolation in cell culture and earlier categorization of viral agents retrieved in cultures of SAR2-CoV specimens, the CDC recommends that this task should be conducted in a BSL-3 laboratory while adopting BSL-3 practices, mainly comprising fit-tested N95 respirators or powered air-purifying respirators [37] (Figure 1).

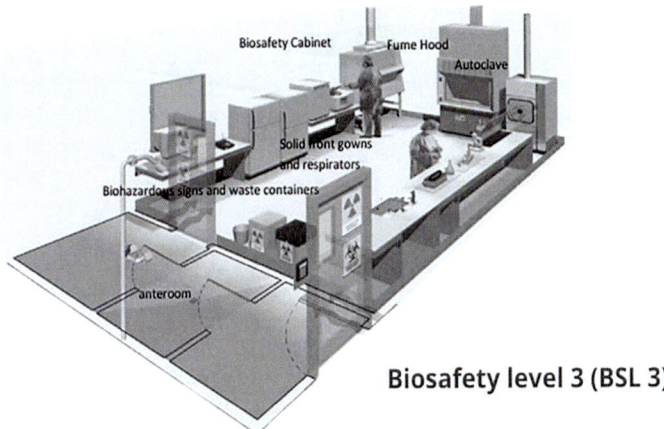

Figure 7.1: Biosafety level 3 biocontainment [38].

Generally, during work within the laboratory, all health care personnel should be given appropriate personal protective equipment (PPE), and techniques for the procurement, transportation and handling of samples should be accessible in written form [36, 39]. All staff members should be trained to adopt proper safety measures, including PPE and the correct use of the mask. A triple-layered surgical mask is enough for all non-aerosol generating processes, whereas N95 or FFP2 masks must be used when conducting aerosol-generating mechanisms. It should be emphasized that the masks should not be allowed to hang from the neck, and they should be changed after 6 hours, or as soon as they become wet or moist. Disposable masks should never be used again and discarded immediately after use in the covered yellow bin, assuming they are potentially infected with medical waste [40, 41].

Doffing is the utmost contaminated procedure and must be conducted in a negative pressure room. Removal of PPE must only be done while exiting the laboratory, and their proper disposal should be made necessary in suitable biomedical trash bins. All PPE must be applied as per doffing guidelines, and hand hygiene should be conducted, even in between the doffing process. Any laboratory personnel who develop symptoms resembling COVID-19 patients should immediately report to their concerned medical authorities. Moreover, additional precautions should be taken for staff that are elderly or have a history of cardiovascular disease, diabetes mellitus, chronic respiratory disorder, malignancy, or on chemo or radiotherapy [41, 42].

The WHO guidelines suggest that all specimens received for histopathology and cytopathology should be considered possibly infectious, and particular regulations were recommended to minimize the exposure to the virus. The histological protocol for these samples comprises separate storage and grossing areas, and adequate sanitation of the external and internal compartments of both the cabinet and hood, before and after use. The formalin fixation for 48 hours must be maintained in an allocated fume cabinet, grossing of the samples in a committed, certified, class II biological safety hood, and disposal of sharps and other materials according to daily practices adopted for hospital waste management. These biosafety measures should be conducted by trained technicians and medical staff wearing proper personal protective equipment (PPE) in a laboratory room with a controlled ventilation system that maintains inward directional airflow [43].

In the case of COVID-19 infection, the cytopathology biosafety approach comprises a combination of education and supply, environmental safety, transportation, handling and processing, and specific endorsement of rapid on-site evaluations (ROSE) [44]. Various routinely processed cytology samples are believed to be infectious, including pleural effusion, bronchoalveolar lavage, bronchoalveolar washing, transbronchial needle aspiration, and sputum. To reduce the steps resulting in aerosol formation or the creation of droplets, it is necessary to follow ROSE and reassess to eliminate undue exposure. Following BSL-II guidelines by the WHO, routine specimens should be processed. According to the WHO guidelines, all samples should be placed in suitable containers, conveyed at 2°C to 8°C, and stored at 2°C to 8°C (short term) or −70°C (long term; on a dry-ice pack) till laboratory testing is done. To avoid the droplets/aerosols while preparing smears, heat fixing, or staining, a BSL-II cabinet (BSC) should be used [45]. Though the same protocols are utilized for cytology samples, yet for most of the preparations, a relatively low alcohol concentration is used, so the procedure alterations for cytology should be more meticulous than for histology samples.

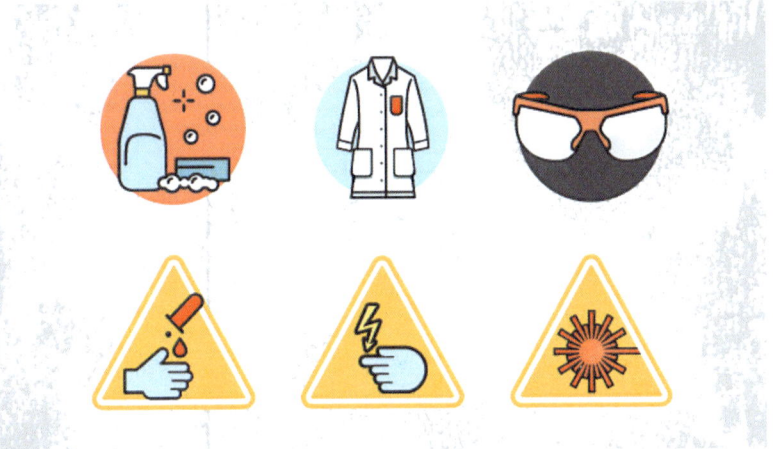

Figure 7.2: Laboratory safety rules and guidelines [46].

Tissue Specimens of COVID 19 in the Pathology Laboratory

For diagnosing and screening patients with COVID-19 pneumonia, early respiratory tract sample collection becomes the foremost challenge for any laboratory personnel. The patients presenting to the laboratory for diagnosis are usually at the stage where they have revealed increased viral loads in their respiratory tract specimens. While taking an adequate nasopharyngeal or an oropharyngeal swab, close interaction with the patients requires strict adherence to infection prevention and control guidelines through the use of gloves, PPE, face masks, face shields, and ideally, the sample should be taken in a reverse-pressure ventilated room or open air space. Secondly, only personnel with demonstrated capabilities should perform all procedures based on risk assessment. The less risky samples include sputum, bronchial washing, or bronchoalveolar lavage. Even having the highest viral loads still saves the personnel from direct physical exposure to the patient during direct nasal or oral sampling. However, utmost care should be sought for non-propagative diagnostic work when steering procedures with an unusual probability of generating aerosol or droplets. The specimens must be transported to the laboratories in guanidinium-based inactivating agents that cause inactivation of viable coronavirus [47, 48]. For viral DNA extraction, ideally, self-enclosed systems incorporating nucleic acid extraction, amplification, and detection, such as

ID NOW (Abbott, San Diego, CA), Cobas Liat (Roche Molecular Systems, Pleasanton, CA), and GeneXpert (Cepheid, Sunnyvale, CA), become highly useful [49-51]. In most developing countries, point-of-care testing for local hospitals and clinics lacks sufficient funds and equipment to work under BSL-3 conditions. In such settings, the role of local health care regulatory bodies becomes vital for implementing strict legislation and policies for the local laboratories ensuring COVID-19 testing, which must be carried out in standard approved laboratories [52].

The competitive laboratory environment for short-turnaround-time (STAT) tests becomes another challenge for the laboratory owners, managers, and staff working there. Most state-of-the-art laboratories offer safe, simple, and fast assays with reports issued within 24-48 hours [53]. With the establishment of new COVID treatment and management centers worldwide, these short turnaround times are considered imperative for timely patient management and infection control decisions, thus meaning that these laboratories are running 24/7 to cater to hospitals, clinics, patients, and patients' travel industries. The other side of the story reveals that at the hospitals and clinics, the routine/elective surgeries, and procedures came to a halt during the pandemic, significantly reducing the number of routine non-emergency samples registering at the laboratories. Due to the heavy turnover of the SARS-Cov-2 testing, the turnaround time of the routine diagnostic tests, including biopsies and serology, suffered delays of weeks, and even months, in some regions of the world. Many laboratories had to outsource their emergency testing to issue reports on the urgent requests by physicians and surgeons [54, 55].

During the pandemic, most professions all over the world have shifted to work-from-home mode. On the contrary, the laboratory staff have had to work double their usual time. However, staff strength was also increased within most laboratories' existing physical space to handle the increasing workload, which was greater than the in-house analysis capacity. The lack of sleep and rest, and minimal interaction with their families during heavy workloads adversely affects the immune system of laboratory workers. It increases psychological pressure leading to poor health. According to the latest CDC guidelines, frequent and appropriate testing facilities for the laboratory workers engaged in SARS-CoV-2 testing must be available for timely diagnosis and management. The expanded use of technology, including digital pathology, has become a fairy-tale story for developing economies.

Moreover, the laboratories, especially in developing countries, also suffered a critical halt in importing and delivering the chemicals/reagents kits and consumables for routine diagnostics and research purposes. Long waiting times had to be faced when procuring corona-related testing and research reagents; however, intensive management of medicines and supplies remained uninterrupted.

The fulfillment of external quality control, quality assurance practices, audits, and reviews of the laboratory workflow is another challenge in running laboratories, due to the heavy engagement of staff in COVID testing. Documentation and data compilation, with weekly or monthly report generation, seemed like an essential activity due to the demand and pressure from governments for the statistical output.

Simultaneously, professional development activities, hands-on training, and workshops remained interrupted throughout the year. Most doctors, pathologists, and staff utilized online learning and training tools for their best practice. This virtual education and training remains insufficient for junior pathologists and laboratory workers.

Autopsy Handling During COVID-19

Coroners and autopsy pathologists have become indispensable during this pandemic as necropsy and cadaver lung examination, with other death investigations, has become the mainstay for studying the pathobiological response of SARS-CoV-2 in the human pulmonary system. Also, detection and localization of the virus within the human lungs became possible only after gross and microscopic evaluation of the lung tissues (Figure 7.3).

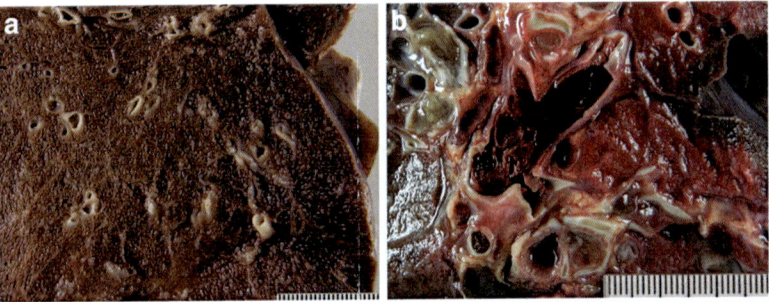

Figure 7.3: Gross Images of a COVID-19 lung with interstitial edema and congestion; b) pulmonary embolism in COVID-19 [56].

It is generally reported that active viruses can be isolated from the cadavers of SARS up to 175 hours after death, signifying that the cadaver examiners may directly acquire the virus if the biosafety precautions are not rigorously practiced [57]. Appropriate legislation and guidelines must be followed, including establishing the facility at a reasonable distance from the main hospital or clinic to avoid exposure of other staff and the public. It is advisable to conduct the post-mortem examination with a restricted number of examiners to reduce the likelihood of infection. Spraying/wiping with 75% v/v ethanol, or exposure to ultraviolet for at least one hour, is recommended for some devices, such as a camera or digital record, that are not appropriate for disinfection by disinfectant or ultraviolet [58]. Suitable disposal of the greywater and waste must be appropriately managed. Reusable instruments and equipment must be adequately disinfected. All the specimens must be transported in recommended preservatives and transport media.

Conclusion

The responses of governments and institutions while facing the challenges of COVID-19 are the limpid proof of their political, financial, and legislative authority. In the present era, it is each individual's fundamental right to be given protection against communicable diseases, particularly those that are alarmingly fatal for public health. This protection must be available to the masses at all levels, regardless of gender, race, and economic status. The health sector all over the world transformed its approach towards patient care and end-point diagnostics. A dramatic surmount in the provision of intensive care facilities, protective gear, emergency medicines, RT-PCR diagnostics, and management of terminally ill patients was noted with time. Through ongoing and effective media awareness campaigns and digital education services, frontline health care workers' physical, psychological, and emotional maladies stayed efficiently restrained. The young and old, juniors and seniors, trained and lesser skilled – all frontline workers were ready to fight the pandemic despite the meager support from governments and international health care funding agencies. A massive research fund was released and utilized throughout the world to provide clues to the practical and authentic diagnostic, management, and digital health solutions for SARS-CoV-2 infection. Though, at the preliminary levels, the results of Phase I-IV clinical trials throughout the world provided a breakthrough in the development and approval of effective COVID-19 vaccines for marketing and use by the general public.

Nevertheless, serious gaps in the response to the disease and to coping with a future pandemic of similar or graver nature still exist even in highly developed economies and health care systems. At this stage, it is pretty premature to assume the longer-term behavior, severity, and tenacity of COVID-19, but the lessons learned so far will prove to be a turning point for all health care systems throughout the world. Health care workers shall remain on the frontline against the various challenges that the COVID-19 contagion is putting forward, day by day. Hence, preparedness for public health safety measures through capitalizing on novel preventive, diagnostic, and management tools for the sustenance, well-being, and protection of health care workers, and the public at large, should be the priority goal of every country in the world.

References

1. Perez HR, Beyrouty M, Bennett K, Manwell LB, Brown RL, Linzer M, Schwartz MD. Chaos in the clinic: characteristics and consequences of practices perceived as chaotic. J Healthc Qual (JHQ). 2017 Jan 1;39(1):43-53.

2. Pozzer A, Dominici F, Haines A, Witt C, Münzel T, Lelieveld J. Regional and global contributions of air pollution to the risk of death from COVID-19. Cardiovasc Res. 2020;116(14):2247-53.

3. Contini D, Costabile F. Does Air Pollution Influence COVID-19 Outbreaks? Atmosphere. 2020;11(4):377. https://doi.org/10.3390/atmos11040377.

4. Frontera A, Cianfanelli L, Vlachos K, Landoni G, Cremona G. Severe air pollution links to higher mortality in COVID-19 patients: The "double-hit" hypothesis. J Infect. 2020;81(2):255-9.

5. Arumugam M, Menon B, Narayan SK. Ambient temperature and COVID-19 incidence rates: An opportunity for. Emerg Microbes Infect. 2020;9(1).

6. Briz-Redón Á, Serrano-Aroca Á. The effect of climate on the spread of the COVID-19 pandemic: A review of findings and statistical and modeling techniques. Progress in Physical Geography: Earth Environ. 2020;44(5):591-604. https://doi.org/10.1177%2F0309133320946302.

7. Ahmadi M, Sharifi A, Dorosti S, Ghoushchi SJ, Ghanbari N. Investigation of effective climatology parameters on COVID-19 outbreak in Iran. Sci Total Environ. 2020;729:138705.

8. Ozili PK, Arun T. Spillover of COVID-19: Impact on the Global Economy. https://dx.doi.org/10.2139/ssrn.3562570.[Last accessed on 2020 Aug 20].

9. Lambert H, Gupte J, Fletcher H, Hammond L, Lowe N, Pelling M, et al. COVID-19 as a global challenge: towards an inclusive and sustainable future. Lancet Planetary Health. 2020;4(8):e312-14.

10. Diogenes AN, Tedesco DG. A simple stochastic model for the SARS-CoV-2 Epidemic curve. Therm Eng. 2020;19(1):113-8. http://dx.doi.org/10.5380/reterm.v19i1.76443.

11. Wu X, Nethery R, Sabbath M, Braun D, Dominici F. Air pollution and COVID-19 mortality in the United States: Strengths and limitations of an ecological regression analysis. Sci Adv. 2020;6(45):eabd4049. https://doi.org/10.1126/sciadv.abd4049.

12. Kan HD, Chen B-H, Fu CW, Yu S-Z, Mu LN. Relationship between ambient air pollution and daily mortality of SARS in Beijing. Biomed Environ Sci. 2005;18(1):1-4.

13. Comunian S, Dongo D, Milani C Palestini P. Air pollution and Covid-19: the role of particulate matter in the spread and increase of Covid-19's morbidity and mortality. Intern J Environ Res Public Health. 2020;17(12):4487. https://doi.org/10.3390/ijerph17124487.

14. Sizhe H, Rongshuai W, Yunyun W, Junchao Z, Youyou Z, Chuhuai G, et al. COVID-19: A challenge for forensic and pathological researchers. J Forensic Sci Med. 2020;6(2):58-62.

15. Borasio GD, Gamondi C, Obrist M, Jox R. COVID-19: decision making and palliative care. Swiss medical weekly. 2020 Mar 24;150(1314). https://doi.org/10.4414/smw.2020.20233.

16. Corless IB, Nardi D, Milstead JA, Larson E, Nokes KM, Orsega S, Kurth AE, Kirksey KM, Woith W. Expanding nursing's role in responding to global pandemics 5/14/2018. Nurs Outlook. 2018 Jul 1;66(4):412-5. https://doi.org/10.1016/j.outlook.2018.06.003.

17. Crimi C, Carlucci A. Challenges for the female healthcare workers during the COVID-19 pandemic: the need for protection beyond the mask. Pulmonol. 2021 Jan 1;27(1):1-3.

18. Pappa S, Giannakoulis VG, Papoutsi E, Katsaounou P. Author reply–Letter to the editor "The challenges of quantifying the psychological burden of COVID-19 on healthcare workers". Brain Behav Immun. 2020 Jan 1; 92: 209-210. Available online from https://www.ncbi.nlm.nih.gov/pmc/articles/PMC7836696/. [Last accessed on 2021 Feb 11].

19. Rossi R, Socci V, Pacitti F, Di Lorenzo G, Di Marco A, Siracusano A, Rossi A. Mental health outcomes among frontline and second-line health care workers during the coronavirus disease 2019 (COVID-19) pandemic in Italy. JAMA network open. 2020 May 1;3(5):e2010185. https://doi:10.1001/jamanetworkopen.2020.10185.

20. Rahman A, Plummer V. COVID-19 related suicide among hospital nurses; case study evidence from worldwide media reports. Psychiatry Res. 2020 Sep 1;291:113272.

21. Lu X, Xu S. Important role of emergency department doctors after the outbreak of covid-19 in China. Emerg Med J. 2020 Jun 1;37(6):334. http://dx.doi.org/10.1136/emermed-2020-209633.

22. American Hospital Association. Hospitals and Health Systems Face Unprecedented Financial Pressures Due to COVID-19. Hospitals and Health Systems Face Unprecedented Financial Pressures Due to COVID-19 | AHA. Available online from https://www.aha.org/guidesreports/2020-05-05-hospitals-and-health-systems-face-unprecedented-financial-pressures-due. [Last accessed on 2021 Feb 12].

23. Sterling MR, Tseng E, Poon A, Cho J, Avgar AC, Kern LM, Ankuda CK, Dell N. Experiences of home health care workers in New York City during the coronavirus disease 2019 pandemic: a qualitative analysis. JAMA Intern Med. 2020 Nov 1;180(11): https://1453-9. doi:10.1001/jamainternmed.2020.3930.

24. Al Thobaity A, Alamri S, Plummer V, Williams B. Exploring the necessary disaster plan components in Saudi Arabian hospitals. Intern J Disaster Risk Reduct. 2019 Dec 1;41:101316. https://doi.org/10.1016/j.ijdrr.2019.101316.

25. Dami F, Yersin B, Hirzel AH, Hugli O. Hospital disaster preparedness in Switzerland. Swiss medical weekly. 2014;144 :w14032. https://doi:10.4414/smw.2014.14032.

26. Guyot K, Sawhill IV. Telecommuting will likely continue long after the pandemic. Brookings Institution. 2020 Apr 6;6. Available online from https://www.brookings.edu/blog/up-front/2020/04/06/telecommuting-will-likely-continue-long-after-the-pandemic/. [Last accessed on 2021 Feb 10].

27. Bilawar PB. Lockdown period and information sources. Intern J Eng Res. 2020; 7 (6).

28. Dasa M, Bhuyanb C, Shahnaz SF. COVID-19 Pandemic-induced Teaching-Learning Experiences: Some Realities from Assam (India). Int. J Innov Creativity Chang. 2020; 14: 353-76.

29. Farooq F, Rathore FA, Mansoor SN. Challenges of online medical education in Pakistan during COVID-19 pandemic. J Coll Physicians Surg Pak. 2020 Jun 1;30(6):67-9. https://doi.org/10.29271/jcpsp.2020. Suppl.S67.

30. Gaur U, Majumder MA, Sa B, Sarkar S, Williams A, Singh K. Challenges and opportunities of preclinical medical education: COVID-19 crisis and beyond. SN Compr Clin Med. 2020 Sep 22:1-6. https://doi.org/10.1007/s42399-020-00528-1.

31. Rajab MH, Gazal AM, Alkattan K. Challenges to online medical education during the COVID-19 pandemic. Cureus. 2020 Jul;12(7): e8966. https://doi.org/10.7759/cureus.8966.

32. Adedoyin OB, Soykan E. Covid-19 pandemic and online learning: the challenges and opportunities. Interactive Learning Environments. 2020 Sep 3:1-3. https://doi.org/10.1080/10494820.2020.1813180.

33. Goh PS, Sandars J. A vision of the use of technology in medical education after the COVID-19 pandemic. MedEdPublish. 2020 Mar 26;9. https://doi.org/10.15694/mep.2020.000049.1.

34. Sizhe H, Rongshuai W, Yunyun W, Junchao Z, Youyou Z, Chuhuai G, et al. COVID-19: A challenge for forensic and pathological researchers. J Forensic Sci Med. 2020;6(2):58-62.

35. Lamas NJ, Esteves S, Alves JR, Costa FE, Tente D, Fonseca P, et al. The anatomic pathology laboratory adjustments in the era of COVID-19 pandemic: the experience of a laboratory in a Portuguese central hospital. Ann Diagn Pathol. 2020;48:151560. https://doi.org/10.1016/j. anndiagpath.2020.151560.

36. World Health Organization (WHO). Laboratory biosafety guidance related to coronavirus disease 2019 (COVID-19): interim guidance, Feb 12, 2020. World Health Organization; 2020. Available online from https://apps.who.int/iris/handle/10665/332076. [Last accessed on 2020 Aug 20].

37. Sick PG, 2020. Interim Laboratory Biosafety Guidelines for Handling and Processing Specimens Associated with Coronavirus Disease 2019 (COVID-19). 31 March 2020 ed. Available online from https://stacks. cdc.gov/view/cdc/86282. [Last accessed on 2020 June 10].

38. World Health Organization (WHO). Laboratory biosafety manual: World Health Organization; 2020. Available online at https://apps.who. int/iris/handle/10665/332076. [Last accessed on 2020 June 10].

39. Iwen PC, Stiles KL, Pentella MA. Safety considerations in the laboratory testing of specimens suspected or known to contain the severe acute

respiratory syndrome coronavirus 2 (SARS-CoV-2). Am J Clin Pathol. 2020;153(5):567-70. https://doi.org/10.1093/ajcp/aqaa047.

40. Ferioli M, Cisternino C, Leo V, Pisani L, Palange P, Nava S. Protecting healthcare workers from SARS-CoV-2 infection: practical indications. Eur Respir Rev. 2020;29(155).

41. Misra V, Agrawal R, Kumar H, Kar A, Kini U, Poojary A, et al. Guidelines for various laboratory sections given COVID-19: Recommendations from the Indian Association of Pathologists and Microbiologists. Indian J Pathol Microbiol. 2020;63(3):350-7.

42. Cook T. Personal protective equipment during the coronavirus disease (COVID) 2019 pandemic–a narrative review. Anesthesia. 2020;75(7):920-7. https://doi.org/10.1111/anae.15071.

43. Rossi ED, Fadda G, Mule A, Zannoni GF, Rindi G. Cytologic and histologic samples from patients infected by the novel coronavirus 2019 SARS-CoV-2: An Italian institutional experience focusing on biosafety procedures. Cancer Cytopathol. 2020;128(5):317-20.

44. Chen CC, Chi CY. Biosafety in preparing and processing cytology specimens with potential coronavirus (COVID-19) infection: Perspectives from Taiwan. Cancer Cytopathol. 2020;128(5):309-16. https://doi.org/10.1002/cncy.22280.

45. Pambuccian SE. The COVID-19 pandemic: implications for the cytology laboratory. Journal of the American Society of Cytopathology. 2020;9(3):202-11. https://doi.org/10.1016/j.jasc.2020.03.001.

46. Manager L, 2017. Lab Safety Rules and Guidelines. Available online from https://www.labmanager.com/lab-health-and-safety/science-laboratory-safety-rules-guidelines-5727.

47. Tang Y-W, Schmitz JE, Persing DH, Stratton CW. Laboratory diagnosis of COVID-19: current issues and challenges. J Clin Microbiol. 2020;58(6). https://doi.org/10.1128/JCM.00512-20.

48. Burton J, Easterbrook L, Pitman J, Anderson D, Roddy S, Bailey D, et al. The effect of a non-denaturing detergent and a guanidinium-based inactivation agent on the viability of Ebola virus in mock clinical serum samples. J Virol Methods. 2017;250:34-40. https://doi.org/10.1016/j.jviromet.2017.09.020.

49. Kanwar N, Michael J, Doran K, Montgomery E, Selvarangan R. Comparison of the ID Now influenza A & B 2, Cobas influenza A/B, and Xpert Xpress Flu point-of-care nucleic acid amplification tests for influenza A/B virus detection in children. J Clin Microbiol. 2020;58(3):e01611-19. https://doi.org/10.1128/JCM.01611-19.

50. Granato PA, Hansen G, Herding E, Chaudhuri S, Tang S, Garg SK, et al. Performance comparison of the Cobas Liat and Cepheid GeneXpert systems for Clostridium difficile detection. PLoS One. 2018;13(7):e0200498. https://doi.org/10.1371/journal.pone.0200498.

51. Wang H, Deng J, Tang Y-W. Profile of the Alere I Influenza A & B assay: a pioneering molecular point-of-care test. Expert Rev Mol Diagn. 2018;18(5):403-9.

52. Mourya DT, Yadav PD, Majumdar TD, Chauhan DS, Katoch VM. Establishment of biosafety level-3 (BSL-3) laboratory: important criteria to consider while designing, constructing, commissioning & operating the facility in the Indian setting. Indian J Med Res. 2014;140(2):171-83. Available online from https://www.ncbi.nlm.nih.gov/pmc/articles/PMC4216491/.

53. Pati HP, Singh G. Turnaround time (TAT): difference in concept for laboratory and clinician. Indian J Hematol Blood Transfus. 2014;30(2):81-4. https://doi.org/10.1007/s12288-012-0214-3.

54. Meredith JW, High KP, Freischlag JA. Preserving elective surgeries in the COVID-19 pandemic and the future. JAMA. 2020;324(17):1725-6. https://doi.org/10.1001/jama.2020.19594.

55. Tan SS, Yan B, Saw S, Lee CK, Chong AT, Jureen R, et al. Practical laboratory considerations amidst the COVID-19 outbreak: early experience from Singapore. 2020. Report No.: 0021-9746. Available online from http://dx.doi.org/10.1136/jclinpath-2020-206563. [Last accessed on 2020 Oct 15].

56. Mohanty SK, Satapathy A, Naidu MM, Mukhopadhyay S, Sharma S, Barton LM, et al. Severe acute respiratory syndrome coronavirus-2 (SARS-CoV-2) and coronavirus disease 19 (COVID-19)–anatomic pathology perspective on current knowledge. Diagn Pathol. 2020;15(1):1-17. https://doi.org/10.1186/s13000-020-01017-8.

57. Sizhe H, Rongshuai W, Yunyun W, Junchao Z, Youyou Z, Chuhuai G, et al. COVID-19: A challenge for forensic and pathological researchers. J Forensic Sci Med. 2020;6(2):58-61. https://doi.org/10.4103/jfsm.jfsm_27_20.

58. World Health Organization (WHO). Water, sanitation, hygiene, and waste management for the COVID-19 virus: interim guidance, Apr 23 2020. World Health Organization; 2020. Available online from https://apps.who.int/iris/handle/10665/331499. [Last accessed on 2020 June 22].

COVID-19 Pandemic and Human Rights: Challenges and Responsibilities

Chapter 08

Tehreem Sultan

Abstract

Severe Acute Respiratory Syndrome (SARS-CoV-2), recognized as the COVID-19 Pandemic, swiftly took over the entire world and caused great public health and socioeconomic harm. To reduce the spreading and transmission of SARS-CoV-2, over 100 states globally implemented policies of partial or complete lockdown measures, which form the basis of human rights in this lockdown. This was restricted by necessity for freedom of movement and, in the process, freedom to enjoy many other human rights. Due to this unpredictable turn of events, the travel system had been paralyzed, and approximately 3 billion people were stranded in their homes. Furthermore, a large majority of people also lost their jobs orwere furloughed. This pandemic led to devastating health concerns and added to the psychological distress and mental health issues in society. Therefore, there is a pressing need to shed light on protecting every individual's human rights, including adopting a non-discrimination policy, transparency, and respect for human dignity in every country. Human Rights are essential in shaping the pandemic response. It is vital to ensure policies provide equal health services and assist in accommodating individuals back to their positions in society, both personally and professionally.

Keywords: COVID-19 pandemic, SARS-CoV-2, Human Rights, Challenges and Responses

1. Introduction

On December 29 2019, Wuhan, in the Hubei province of China, experienced an outbreak of pneumonia from a novel coronavirus, the Severe Acute Respiratory Syndrome Coronavirus 2 (SARS-CoV-2). SARS-CoV-2, also known as the COVID-19 pandemic, swiftly took over the entire world and caused great public health and socioeconomic harm [1]. The World Health Organisation declared it as a global pandemic and a high-priority emergency. By February 26 2021, it had affected 216 countries, 112,649,317 people resulting in 2,501,229 deaths (2.22%) worldwide [2]. The COVID-19 pandemic hit these countries the hardest: China, the United States of America, India, Brazil, the Russian Federation, the United

Kingdom, France, Italy, Spain, Germany, etc. The majority of the countries are from America and Europe [WHO 2021] (Figure 8.1).

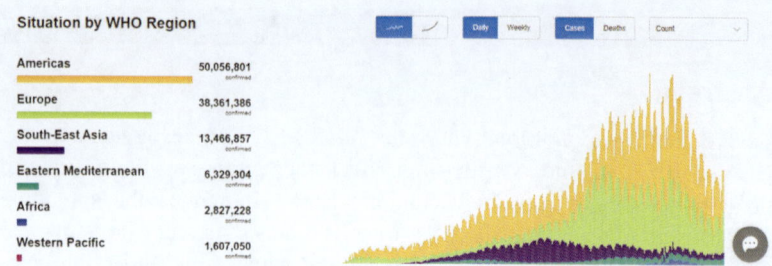

Figure 8.1: A worldwide number of cases due to SARS-CoV-2 infection. World Health Organization Report [February 26, 2021 [2].

As of March 2020, over 100 states implemented partial or complete lockdown measures to minimize the spread of the coronavirus. Due to this unforeseen situation, the travel system had been paralyzed, and about 3 billion people were stranded in their homes [3]. While there is no doubt that these lockdown measures were taken to minimize the transmission of this deadly contagious disease, we also cannot simply neglect the adverse impact of self-isolation and quarantine on public health, which is not limited to psychological distress and mental health issues, including depression, anxiety, stress [4].

The COVID-19 pandemic rose to the level of a public health threat that could justify imposing restrictions on certain human rights, such as those that result from the imposition of quarantine or limiting freedom of movement. Taking this into careful consideration, special attention is required to protect every individual's human rights, including non-discrimination, transparency, and respect for human dignity in every country. Human Rights are essential in shaping the pandemic response, and adopting extensive lockdown measures could breach the rights under Article 8 of the European Convention on Human Rights [5]. This is also strongly supported by the constitution of various countries, which lies upon the fundamental right of "liberty" for everyone [6, 7]. Thus, measures need to be taken to mitigate any consequences of the violation of human rights.

On March 16 2020, the Office of the United Nations High Commissioner for Human Rights confirmed that states must not abuse emergency measures in order to suppress human rights. The COVID-19 outbreak emergency measures should not be used to target particular groups of individuals or minority groups in the individual nations. The constraints taken in response to the COVID-19 pandemic must be motivated by legitimate public health objectives [8]. This chapter highlights the various international dimensions of human rights to the COVID-19 pandemic and the challenges worldwide.

2. International Human Rights Law in the COVID-19 Pandemic

The world is facing an unprecedented crisis. The first case of SARS-CoV-2 infection was identified on December 29 2019, in Wuhan, China. The SARS-CoV-2 virus does not respect state borders or regions and swiftly spread across the globe through numerous travel modes. The World Health Organization declared the outbreak a Public Health Emergency of International Concern in January 2020 and a pandemic in March 2020 [2].

The international dimensions of human rights are particularly relevant to the present ongoing pandemic and its allied situations. Guaranteeing human rights under the International Covenant on Civil and Political Rights [9] and protecting these rights while ensuring the priority is to save lives poses a challenge for every country in the world, to differing degrees [9]. States across the globe have taken measures to combat COVID-19. These measures, including lockdowns, quarantines, and the provision of treatment in hospitals, have engaged critical human rights concerns. Therefore, the public health crisis is becoming an economic and social crisis coupled with a protection and human rights crisis, all rolled into one. The protection of human rights globally requires mutual agreements and international solidarity. Recognizing that states have different resources and norms, human rights laws and guidance can provide a basis for assessing how well governments' measures promote people's human rights while protecting public health [10].

The five fundamental human rights principles are particularly relevant to pandemic responses [a] equality and non-discrimination, [b] participation, [c] proportionality, [d] human dignity and care, and [e] rights to freedom of expression, assembly, and information [10]. Equality and non-discrimination forms of discrimination cause inequality, and are relevant to the coronavirus outbreak.

3. Freedom of Movement in the COVID-19 Pandemic

Traveling during the COVID-19 pandemic is posing an immense challenge for airlines and transportation, including trains, buses, airports, travelers, health authorities, and governments. The COVID-19 health crisis affected millions of people attempting to travel to their destinations, including their homes, workplaces, schools, and universities. Due to this travel ban and restriction on movement, people could not avail themselves of their annual vacations, family visits, and business trips. The COVID-19 outbreak has markedly affected the travel, tourism, hotel, and food industries and caused an employment crisis [11, 12].

Mainly focusing on Europe, the arrival of tourists in European countries markedly decreased by 38%-68% in 2020. This situation placed 6.6 to 11.7 million jobs at risk of reduced working hours or permanent job losses in 2020. These factors led to a change in living standards, impaired the quality of life and human behavior, raising concerns about psychological illnesses and economic losses. Moreover, the economic indicators are allied with a decline in household income due to unemployment or a reduction in working hours [13]. To mitigate the spread of the coronavirus, governments throughout the world have introduced emergency measures that constrain individual freedoms and have imposed domestic and international travel bans. The literature has reported that travel restrictions can delay the initial spread of COVID-19, with infection prevention and control measures being essential to minimize the transmission [14]. Furthermore, researchers concluded that "travel restrictions are most useful in the early and late phase of an epidemic" and "restrictions of travel from Wuhan, unfortunately, came too late to prevent the transmission." However, the literature also suggests that the impact of border closures is temporary and limited, and therefore, alternative measures must be implemented to limit the spread of COVID-19 [15].

In another study, it has been demonstrated that travel limitations effectively contained the COVID-19 epidemic during the epidemic peak in China. The literature also supports the hypothesis that the effectiveness of travel bans is applied to countries with high disease prevalence [16]. On the contrary, Shi et al., 2020 [17] demonstrated that travel restrictions were not sufficient to prevent the global spread of SARS-CoV-2; further research should also consider travel by land and sea. Their study findings highlight the importance of strengthening local capacities for disease monitoring and control. However, strategies to restrict the traveling network have a significant economic and social impact [18].

These travel bans and the restricting quarantine steps confirm the haphazard and disorganized regulations being imposed. Moreover, this travel ban lockdown is challenging to sustain in developing nations, especially amongst societies where traveling is essential for work purposes. In these situations, fundamental rights are severely impaired and violated since individuals cannot carry out their everyday work. Therefore, this directly imposes a duty on states to ensure everyone has access to food, basic living needs, coronavirus testing, and treatment facilities under the 30 Articles set out by the Universal Declaration of Human Rights (UDHR) [19]. Under Article 14, equality and non-discrimination are core human rights that apply at all times, but this pandemic clearly shows why inequality and discriminatory practices are unacceptable, and hurt everyone. We cannot afford to leave anyone behind in fighting the pandemic. The COVID-19 pandemic is revealing underlying structural inequalities that are causing certain groups to be disproportionately affected. The way COVID-19 is hitting specific communities, especially the marginalized, demonstrated this.

Moreover, there must be no patterns of discriminatory behavior that can affect the accessibility of people for testing and treatment objectives. The state must also ensure that financial barriers do not prevent people from accessing testing and treatment for COVID-19. Moreover, governmental officials confirm that the COVID-19 allied health crisis and quarantine crisis have not become human rights crises. The authorities must attempt to return to a normal lifestyle and avoid excessive use of emergency powers for an indefinitely long period [7].

4. The Lockdown Measures and Human Rights Violations

COVID-19 has diverse biological and prevalence characteristics, making it more contagious than earlier pandemics, such as SARS-CoV and MERS-CoV [1]. The highly contagious nature of COVID-19 causes a threatening situation worldwide. Approximately 3.9 billion people are quarantining in their homes [3]. Many states implemented quarantine or isolation policies to contain people and minimize the spread of the disease. The quarantine period included short to medium-term lockdowns, voluntary home restrictions, cancellation of social and public events, and travel restrictions [20]. This situation has created a global public and psychological health crisis. It has also caused stress and changes in learning behaviors as well as deterioration in work performance [21].

Specific nations imposed restrictions with little respect for the rights of citizens. Looking at China, in mid-January, authorities quarantined close to 60 million people in two days to limit transmission from the city of Wuhan in Hubei province, where the virus was first reported. There were numerous incidents reported in Human Rights Watch, where many residents in cities under quarantine expressed difficulties obtaining medical care and other life necessities, and chilling stories have emerged of deaths and illnesses resulting from these lockdown measures [22]. Comparatively, nations like Italy, South Korea, Hong Kong, Taiwan, and Singapore have responded to the outbreak without enacting sweeping restrictions on personal liberty, which is vital to protect human rights [22]. Government strategies must minimize disruption to services and develop contingency services to compensate for the losses during the COVID-19 pandemic [22].

Focusing on the impact the lockdown measures have on mental health, Röhr et al., 2020 [23] reported that quarantine during the COVID-19 outbreaks developed negative health consequences and mental health impairment. In another study, Lei et al., 2020 [24] identified a rising prevalence of anxiety and depression among people quarantined during the COVID-19 outbreak. Brooks et al., [2020] [25] reported adverse psychological effects, including post-traumatic stress symptoms, confusion, and anger due to the COVID-19 outbreak quarantine. The authors observed that long-term quarantine causes fear and frustration, and that inadequate information and financial losses are the leading causes of negative psychological impact.

Similarly, Meo et al., 2020 [21] found that people felt disheartened and depressed. People considered the lockdown an unpleasant experience because of separation from colleagues, friends, and family. Hawryluck et al., 2004 [4] showed a high prevalence of psychological distress, post-traumatic stress disorder (PTSD) (28.9%), and depression (31.2%). Moreover, long-term quarantine was significantly linked with PTSD.

The World Health Organization (WHO) [26] and the Centers for Disease Control and Prevention [27] have published a note on Mental Health and Psycho-Social Support (MHPSS), especially for the elderly, children, and people with disabilities during isolation/quarantine for COVID-19.

5. Close Proximity in Prisons during the COVID-19 Pandemic

COVID-19, like other infectious diseases, poses a higher risk to populations that live close to each other, specifically in prison conditions, jails, immigration detention centers, and residential institutions. Therefore, states have a positive obligation to ensure medical care for those in their custody equivalent to that available to the general population and not deny primary health care and rights to specific individuals. Under the Right to Life (Article 2 ECHR) [28], the state is under a substantive (or operational) duty to protect life concerning vulnerable people under the care of the state, such as those detained by the state in prisons, psychiatric detention and immigration detention facilities [28].

The coronavirus poses significantly more risk to these individuals otherwise deprived of their liberty. Prisons and detention centers are often overcrowded, and social distancing is difficult, if not impossible, to maintain when close to one another. The World Health Organization recognizes this in its guidance on preventing and controlling the outbreak of COVID-19, which states that "people in prisons and other places of detention are not only likely to be more vulnerable to infection with Covid-19, they are also especially vulnerable to human rights violations [29]."

For instance, a public health emergency was declared in the United Kingdom's overcrowded prisons. The emergency protocols reduced the time inmates spent out of their cells to about 30 minutes a day and restricted them to their cells for 23 hours, suspended prison transfers, and forced new arrivals to be quarantined for 14 days. Moreover, with the lack of family visits and rehabilitation services, including education services available, the pandemic has had a significant impact on prisoners, as recognized by the Court of Appeal in the United Kingdom's case of R Manning [30]. Similarly, due to protests in Italy over fears of contagion in overcrowded facilities and against bans on family visits and supervised release during the coronavirus pandemic, authorities have authorized, for the first time, the use of email and Skype for contact between prisoners and their families and for educational purposes, and also announced a plan to release and place under house arrest prisoners with less than 18 months on their sentence [22].

Moreover, severely substandard health care has contributed to the recent deaths of immigrants in the custody of US Immigration and Customs Enforcement. Populations in custody often include older people and people with serious chronic health conditions, meaning they are at greater risk of illness from COVID-19 [31]. The position of care homes is more nuanced, but, arguably, at least some of the steps taken in the context of the Covid-19 pandemic have given rise to sufficient state involvement; hence, as a trigger, its operational duty to secure the right to life of those subject to Deprivation of Liberty Safeguards (DoLS) within care homes. In the circumstances, it is right that Governments' responses to Covid-19 in detention settings should receive particular scrutiny from a human rights perspective. Therefore, while numerous countries ensure they carry out their obligations, greater attention must be given to specific overcrowded places where COVID-19 poses a greater risk to the individuals.

6. COVID-19 Pandemic and Health Care

During the past year of the COVID-19 pandemic, there has been a significant imbalance between the need to treat patients with other severe health diseases and the fundamental rights of COVID-19 patients for receiving treatment. In many countries, the health care officials focused on SARS-CoV-2 infections and neglected other patients suffering from various debilitating diseases. In many countries, the limited health resources raised ethical concerns as well as health issues. The COVID-19 pandemic lockdown phase led health care policymakers to prioritize community safety above individuals' rights. This approach to clinical care management has created stress among health care workers [32]. It ignores ordinary care to deal with the pandemic.

During outbreaks of infectious diseases, the scientific and medical community has to adopt measures regarding prevention, immunization, and antimicrobial treatments to preserve the good of public health. During the COVID-19 pandemic, health care officials worldwide focused on fighting the pandemic, and financial resources were redistributed to provide prevention, detection, and treatment of, as well as recovery from COVID-19 disease. Furthermore, patients who were suffering from other chronic diseases were ignored during the pandemic period. Patients' rights vary all over the world due to various ethics, and cultural and social forms. The problem that emerges is that chronic diseases are underestimated or overlooked. This situation endangers patients' rights to health care providers.

The current COVID-19 pandemic has led health care professionals to adopt mandatory restrictive measurements to treat their patients. The medical community has focused mainly on fighting COVID-19. As a result, patients suffering from other diseases, such as diabetes mellitus, coronary artery diseases, Chronic Obstructive Pulmonary diseases, Tuberculosis, Hepatitis, and malignancy, have had their hospital visits postponed because of fear of infection or have not been followed-up by their concerned physician. This situation endangers the rights of those patients who belong to a subgroup of a vulnerable population. Indeed, health officials must respond effectively to the global threat of COVID-19. However, we must not let it overshadow everything and overlook the needs, personalized therapy, and follow-up of non-infected patients. They have the right to continue to have access to the services of the public health system. Justice is ensuring equity and fairness in how patients are treated. It is a matter of importance to learn from history that the global community cannot afford to repeat past mistakes from previous devastating pandemics by neglecting other patients when battling the inevitable pandemic of COVID-19, or other pandemics in the future [33].

7. SARS-COV-2 Virus Vaccination and Human Rights

Early in the COVID-19 pandemic, it was clear that resources were not unlimited and even resource-rich societies needed to re-think thepriorities of allocating resources. The vaccine delivery systems must go beyond infection and immunity, safety, and efficacy. The health authorities consider the allocation of limited vaccine supplies. During the initial nine months of COVID-19, research data revealed that 33 papers were unsuitable for public use and were retracted or withdrawn [34]. The desire to speedily control the pandemic should not allow acceptance of incompletely vetted research findings. The risks and benefits must be balanced carefully. Many wealthy countries have purchased huge stocks of COVID-19 vaccines, with more than 2 billion doses [Callaway, 2020 [35]; however, developing nations, mainly the developing countries, are far away from this race of getting the vaccination.

There are three main ethical issues related to COVID-19 vaccine allocation. First, it was reported that providing benefit while limiting harm is a universal value and that a vaccine could reduce illness and death while mitigating unemployment, poverty, and educational deprivation. Second, they believe that it is fundamental to prioritize disadvantaged populations, including the medically vulnerable who risk earlier death if infected and subject to socioeconomic deprivation. Third, they suggest that differences of race, gender, and religion should not be considered in simplistic ways that could harm or de-prioritize the disadvantaged population [36].

Viruses do not respect borders. A well-coordinated global approach to developing and distributing COVID-19 vaccines, based on the solidarity of all nations and peoples, is the most effective, sustainable, and moral response to the crisis the world is facing. Access to an essential lifesaving vaccine is a core human rights obligation. Health facilities are the fundamental right of all individuals, and COVID-19 vaccines should be treated as global public goods rather than as marketplace commodities available only to those nations who can afford to pay the price. The availability of vaccines, medicines, health technologies, and health therapies is an essential dimension of the right to health, the right to development, and the right to enjoy the benefits of scientific progress and its applications. On an equal footing with others, everyone is entitled to enjoy access to all the best available applications of scientific progress necessary to enjoy the highest attainable standard of health [37].

The World Health Organization recommends that more prosperous nations ensure that resource-limited countries receive early vaccines [38]. It is hoped that national and international law will serve as a means, rather than as a barrier, to just and equitable distribution of vaccines worldwide [39]. COVID-19 vaccines should be affordable to all and accessible without discrimination. Prioritization of vaccine delivery should be done through transparent protocols and procedures that respect human rights. Private profit should not be prioritized over public health. States have to prevent unreasonably high costs for access to essential medicines and vaccines [40].

8. The Employment Crisis in the COVID-19 Pandemic

The COVID-19 pandemic has negatively impacted global employment and economies and caused an unprecedented crisis to all industries worldwide [41]. Tourism, lodging, and travel businesses are highly sensitive to severe shocks and are affected by these epidemics [42]. In particular, the hotel industry has experienced dramatic sales losses as occupancy rates have dropped, mainly due to social distancing and the drastic decline in the number of tourists [43]. The hotel industry experienced an employment shock earlier than other industries, with a sharp drop in employees and a dramatic rise in the number on temporary leave [43].

The COVID-19 pandemic creates behavioral, psychological, economic, unemployment, and emotional challenges that worsen the outcomes of the pandemic [44]. About 60 million people were pushed into extreme poverty (less than $1.90 or £1.55 per person per day) due to the pandemic, and the recovery of these poor people from this phase may take a long time [45]. The impact of the COVID-19 crisis affected mainly the youth who were highly vulnerable before the problem. Massive job losses and the growing precarity of work are having particularly painful impacts on young people worldwide. The COVID-19 economic crisis, with vast increases in unemployment, results in a significant dislocation of young workers from the labor market [46].

COVID-19 rapidly increased the unemployment rate, decreased hours of work, and labor force participation. The negative impact on labor market outcomes is more significant for men, and younger workers [Béland, et al. 2020] [47]. It has been reported that in European Union (EU) states, the economic situation has worsened, the states are deeply concerned about their financial future, and the COVID crisis is so deep that it will not only affect labor markets in the short and medium term, but it can also substantially change the way the work is organized [48].

It is estimated that over eight million jobs were furloughed in the UK, during which the Government paid up to 80% of the UK median salary, to a maximum of £2,500 [47, 49]. However, recent figures indicate that being furloughed by an employer is associated with poorer mental health, with higher levels of stress and anxiety [50]. These are the multiple factors that directly, or indirectly, harm human rights during the COVID-19 pandemic.

Conclusion

The COVID-19 pandemic swiftly took over the entire world and caused great public health and socioeconomic harm. Worldwide, over 100 states implemented the policies of partial or complete lockdown measures to minimize the spread of COVID-19. Due to this unpredictable turn in events, the travel system has been paralyzed and about 3 billion people were stranded in their homes. A large number of people were removed from their services and became jobless. It has created health and psychological distress, and mental health issues globally.

Moreover, this pandemic ignored those people who suffered from other diseases such as diabetes mellitus, coronary artery disease, chronic obstructive pulmonary diseases, and malignancies to get their health facilities and treatment. Human rights are essential in shaping the pandemic response and adopting the policies to provide equal health services, and bring the people back to their services. Special attention is required to protect every individual's human rights, including non-discrimination, transparency, and respect for human dignity in every country.

References

1. Meo SA, Al-Khlaiwi T, Usmani AM, Meo AS, Klonoff DC, Hoang TD. Biological and Epidemiological Trends in the Prevalence and Mortality due to Outbreaks of Novel Coronavirus COVID-19. J King Saud Univ Sci. 2020 Apr 9. doi: 10.1016/j.jksus.2020.04.004.

2. World Health Organization: Available at: https://www.who.int/emergencies/diseases/novel-coronavirus-2019, cited date Feb 26, 2021.

3. BBC. Available at: https://www.bbc.com/news/world-52103747. Cited date May 1, 2020.

4. Hawryluck L, Gold WL, Robinson1 S, Pogorski S, Galea S, Styra R. SARS control and psychological effects of quarantine, Toronto, Canada. Emerg Infect Dis. 2004 Jul;10(7):1206-1212.

5. European Court of Human Rights: Guide on Article 8 of the European Convention on Human Rights. Available at: https://www.echr.coe.int/Documents/Guide_Art_8_ENG.pdf. Cited date May 07, 2020.

6. The Constitution of the Islamic Republic of Pakistan: Chapter 1 Fundamental Rights. Available at: http://www.pakistani.org/pakistan/constitution/part2.ch1.html. Cited date May 07, 2020.

7. Tehreem Sultan. COVID-19: Quarantine and human rights. J Pak Med Assoc. 2020; 70 (Suppl 3) (5): S157. doi: 10.5455/JPMA.42. doi: https://doi.org/10.5455/JPMA.42

8. United Nations Human Rights: Office of the High Commissioner. Available at: rights.https://www.ohchr.org/EN/NewsEvents/ Pages/DisplayNews.aspx?NewsID=25722. Cited date May 01, 2020.

9. The International Covenant on Civil and Political Rights. Available at https://www.ohchr.org/en/professionalinterest/pages/ccpr.aspx. Cited date February 14, 2021.

10. Oxfam Discussion Paper. COVID-19 and Human rights States' obligations and businesses' responsibilities in responding to the Pandemic. Oxfam GB for Oxfam International. ISBN 978-1-78748-633-1 2020. DOI: 10.21201/2020.6331 Oxfam GB, Oxfam House, John Smith Drive, Cowley, Oxford, OX4 2JY, UK.

11. Santos, A.; Cincera, M. (2018). "Tourism demand, low-cost carriers, and European institutions: The case of Brussels," Journal of Transport Geography, 73:163-171.

12. Milasi, S.; González-Vázquez, I.; and Fernández-Macía, E. (2020). "Telework in the EU before and after the COVID-19: where we were, where we head to", Science for Policy Briefs, JRC120945.

13. International Labor Organization. Global Employment Trends for Youth 2020. Available at:https://www.ilo.org/wcmsp5/groups/public/dgreports/dcomm/ 37648.pdf. Cited January 1, 2020.

14. Chinazzi M, Davis JT, Ajelli M, Gioannini C, Litvinova M, Merler S, Pastore Y Piontti A, Mu K, Rossi L, Sun K, Viboud C, Xiong X, Yu H, Halloran ME, Longini IM Jr, Vespignani A. The effect of travel restrictions on the spread of the 2019 novel coronavirus (COVID-19) outbreak. Science. 2020; 368 (6489): 395-400. doi: 10.1126/science.aba9757.

15. Kang S, Moon J, Kang H, Nam H, Tak S, Cho SI. The Evolving Policy Debate on Border Closure in Korea. J Prev Med Public Health. 2020 Sep;53(5):302-306. doi: 10.3961/jpmph.20.213.

16. Costantino V, Heslop DJ, MacIntyre CR. The effectiveness of full and partial travel bans against COVID-19 spread in Australia for travelers from China during and after the epidemic peak in China. J Travel Med. 2020 Aug 20;27(5):taaa081. doi: 10.1093/jtm/taaa081. PMID: 32453411; PMCID: PMC7313810.

17. Shi S, Tanaka S, Ueno R, Gilmour S, Tanoue Y, Kawashima T, Nomura S, Eguchi A, Miyata H, Yoneoka D. Travel restrictions and SARS-CoV-2 transmission: an effective distance approach to estimate impact. Bull World Health Organ. 2020 August 1;98(8):518-529. doi: 10.2471/BLT.20.255679.

18. The world economy is at risk. Coronavirus: Paris: OECD Economics Department; 2020. Available from: http://www.oecd.org/berlin/publikationen/Interim-Economic-Assessment-2-March-2020.pdf [cited 2020 May 19].

19. Universal Declaration of Human Rights. Available at https://www.un.org/en/universal-declaration-human-rights/. Cited date February 10, 2021.

20. Usher K, Bhullar N, Jackson D. Life in the Pandemic: Social isolation and mental health. J Clin Nurs. 2020 doi:10.1111/jocn.15290.

21. Meo SA, Abukhalaf AA, Alomar AA, Sattar K, Klonoff DC. COVID-19 Pandemic: Impact of Quarantine on Medical Students' Mental Wellbeing and Learning Behaviors. Pak J Med Sci. 2020; 36 (COVID19-S4): S43-S48. doi:10.12669/pjms.36. COVID19-S4.2809.

22. Human Rights Watch, Human Rights Dimensions of COVID-19 Pandemic. Available at https://www.hrw.org/news/2020/03/19/human-rights-dimensions-covid-19-response#_Toc35446580. Cited date February 15, 2021.

23. Röhr S, Müller F, Jung F, Apfelbacher C, Seidler A, Riedel-Heller SG. Psychosocial Impact of Quarantine Measures During Serious Coronavirus Outbreaks: A Rapid Review. Psychiatr Prax. 2020; 47 (4): 179-189.

24. Lei L, Huang X, Zhang S, Yang J, Yang L, Xu M. Comparison of Prevalence and Associated Factors of Anxiety and Depression Among People Affected by versus People Unaffected by Quarantine During the COVID-19 Epidemic in Southwestern China. Med Sci Monit. 2020; 26: e924609.

25. Brooks SK, Webster RK, Smith LE, Woodland L, Wessely S, Greenberg N, Rubin GJ. The psychological impact of quarantine and how to reduce it: a rapid review of the evidence. Lancet. 2020 Mar 14; 395(10227):912-920.

26. World Health Organization (WHO) Geneva: 2020. Coping with stress during the 2019-Nov Outbreak (Handout) Accessed on. https://www.who.int/docs/default-source/coronaviruse/coping-with-stress.pdf. Cited date December 10, 2020.

27. Centers for Disease Control and Prevention, Coping with Stress [CDC] Available at https://www.cdc.gov/coronavirus/2019-ncov/daily-life-coping/managing-stress-anxiety.html. Cited Date Dec30, 2020

28. European Court of Human Rights: Guide on Article 2 of the European Convention on Human Rights. Available at: https://www.echr.coe.int/Documents/Guide_Art_2_ENG.pdf. Cited date February 11, 2021.

29. UK Parliament Publications, The Government's response to COVID-19: human rights implications, Detention. Available at https://publications.parliament.uk/pa/jt5801/jtselect/jtrights/265/26508.htm#_idTextAnchor055. Cited date February 16 2021.

30. England and Wales Court of Appeal (Criminal Division) Decisions, The case of R v Manning. Available at https://www.bailii.org/ew/cases/EWCA/Crim/2020/592.html. Cited Date February 17, 2021.

31. Human Rights Watch, Fatal Consequences Dangerously Substandard Medical Care Immigration. Available at https://www.hrw.org/report/2018/06/20/code-red/fatal-consequences-dangerously-substandard-medical-care-immigration. Cited date February 15, 2021.

32. Ferorelli D, Mandarelli G, Solarino B. Ethical Challenges in Health Care Policy during COVID-19 Pandemic in Italy. Medicine (Kaunas). 2020 Dec 11;56(12):691. doi: 10.3390/medicina56120691. PMID: 33322462; PMCID: PMC7764230.

33. Chrysikos D, Zografos CG, Zografos GC. Thoughts about "other" patients' rights during the COVID-19 Pandemic. J Med Ethics Hist Med. 2020; 13: 11. doi:10.18502/jmehm.v13i11.4386.

34. Bramstedt KA. The carnage of substandard research during the COVID-19 Pandemic: A call for quality. *J Med Ethics* 2020; October 1. doi: 10.1136/medethics-2020-106494.

35. Callaway E. The unequal scramble for coronavirus vaccines—by the numbers. Nature 2020; 584: 506-507.

36. Persad G, Peek ME, Emanuel EJ. Fairly prioritizing groups for access to COVID-19 vaccines. JAMA 2020; September 10. doi: 10.1001/jama.2020.18513.

37. Committee on Economic Social and Cultural Rights (CESCR), General Comment No. 25 (2020) on science and economic, social, and cultural rights. Available at: https://www.ohchr.org/en/hrbodies/cescr/pages/cescrindex.aspx. Cited date January 2, 2020.

38. Subbaraman N. Who gets a COVID vaccine first? Access plans are taking shape. Nature 2020;585:492-493.

39. Phelan AL, Eccleston-Turner M, Rourke M, et al. Legal agreements: Barriers and enablers to global equitable COVID-19 vaccine access. Lancet 2020;396:800-802.

40. Wang EA, Zenilman J, Brinkley-Rubinstein L. Ethical Considerations for COVID-19 Vaccine Trials in Correctional Facilities. JAMA. 2020;324(11):1031–1032. doi:10.1001/jama.2020.15589

41. Jung HS, Jung YS, Yoon HH. COVID-19: The effects of job insecurity on the job engagement and turnover intent of deluxe hotel employees and the moderating role of generational characteristics. Int J Hosp Manag. 2021;92:102703. doi:10.1016/j.ijhm.2020.102703.

42. Chang CL, McAleer M, Ramos V. A charter for sustainable tourism after COVID-19. Sustainability. 2020;12(3671):1–4.

43. Sobieralski J.B. COVID-19 and airline employment: insights from historical uncertainty shocks to the industry. TRIP. 2020;5(100123):1–9

44. Blustein DL, Duffy R, Ferreira JA, Cohen-Scali V, Cinamon RG, Allan BA. Unemployment in the time of COVID-19: A research agenda. J Vocat Behav. 2020;119:103436. doi:10.1016/j.jvb.2020.103436

45. The World Bank defines "extreme poverty" as living on less than $1.90 (£1.55) per person per day. Available at: https://www.bbc.com/news/business-52733706, Cited date January 2, 2021.

46. International Labor Organization. (2020b). Young workers will be hit hard by COVID-19's economic fallout. https://iloblog.org/2020/04/15/young-workers-will-be-hit-hard-by-covid-19s-economic-fallout/ Cited date January 1, 2020.

47. Béland, LP, Brodeur A, Wright T. The short-term economic consequences of COVID-19: exposure to disease, remote work, and government response. IZA Discussion Paper Series 2020; 13159.

48. Eurofound. Living, working, and COVID-19, first findings. 2020. Dublin: Available at https://www.eurofound.europa.eu/publications/report/2020/living-working-and-covid-19. Cited date January 1, 2002.

49. Bell T, Gardiner L, Tomlinson D. Getting Britain Working (Safely) Again: The Next Phase of the Coronavirus Job Retention Scheme. London: Resolution Foundation. 2020.

50. Qualtrics XM. The Other COVID-19 Crisis: Mental Health. Available at: https://www.qualtrics.com/blog/confronting-mental-health/. 2020. Cited date January 1, 2020.

COVID-19 Pandemic: Transition Toward Normalcy

Chapter 09

Sultan Ayoub Meo and David C Klonoff

Abstract

Coronavirus infection is an unpredictable disease course, ranging from asymptomatic to severe, life-threatening infections. Since the appearance of SARS-CoV-2 infection in December 2019, there has been an array of conflicting information on the COVID-19 pandemic, affecting the estimates about when the pandemic will end. So far, there is no development of specific drug therapies. However, the scientific community succeeded in developing Pfizer-BioNTech, Moderna, and a few more vaccines that have been authorized around the world against SARS-CoV-2. These vaccines have been associated with documented humoral immunity lasting for at least 2-4 months. However, at the same time, a few more strains of the virus that are more infectious have been detected in some countries. It is hard to imagine the transition toward normalcy before detailed information on vaccination is provided to many people globally and herd immunity is reached for about 65-75% of the population. COVID-19 will not disappear during this transition but will become a more routine part of the baseline disease burden in society rather than a current pandemic threat. The facts suggest that COVID-19 will possibly end around the end of 2022.

Keywords: SARS-CoV-2, COVID-19 Pandemic, Vaccines, End of the Pandemic.

Introduction

Since the appearance of the first case of SARS-CoV-2 infection in Wuhan, China, in the fourth week of December 2019, the incidence and mortality due to SARS-CoV-2 infection are highly fluctuating from continent to continent and country to country [Meo et al., 2020; Meo et al., 2020 [1, 2]. There is an array of conflicting information on the COVID-19 pandemic, affecting the estimates about when the pandemic will end. It is now harder to imagine the world transitioning towards normalcy and reaching herd immunity before the beginning of 2022. Multiple factors could delay the timelines beyond those described, including no homogeneity in health care systems, great economic and educational differences, cultural and traditional variations, safety issues, early vaccines, supply-chain delays, further mutation, or a shorter duration of vaccine-conferred immunity. Herd immunity can also require vaccines to be timely and effective in reducing transmission of SARS-CoV-2. This is likely, but has not yet been proven at scale [Anderson et al., 2020 [3].

On Feb 13, 2021, worldwide there were 107,686,655 confirmed cases of COVID-19, including 2,368,571 deaths [World Health Organization, 2021] [4].

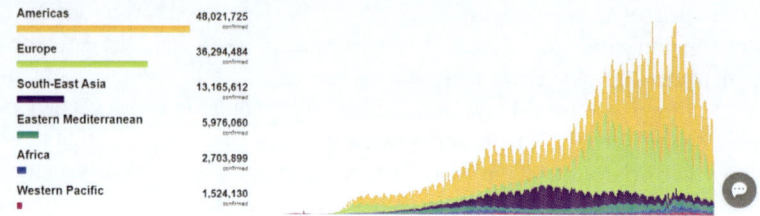

Figure 9.1: Worldwide total number of SARS-CoV-2 cases and deaths [WHO, 2021] [4].

The science community, health officials, policymakers, and the general public collectively fight against this pandemic. However, after more than a year of struggling, the daily cases have, more or less, been gradually increasing. However, the death rate has decreased. There are several possible ways for the transmission of SARS-CoV-2 infection, and person-to-person transmission is proposed as the leading route of infection. The main sources of transmission from human to human are airborne, through respiratory droplets and aerosol particles. Humans produce respiratory droplets of 0.1 to 1000 μm in size. Transmission can be variable based on the droplet size, environment, inertia, gravity, evaporation, and how far emitted droplets and aerosols can travel and stay in the environment. The literature shows that the respiratory droplets with a size of about ~100 μm produced during coughing and sneezing rapidly underwent gravitational settling. These droplets of 100-μm will settle to the ground from 8 feet in 4.6 s, whereas a 1-μm aerosol particle will take about 12 hours to settle in the environment [5].

The current evidence suggests that SARS-CoV-2 infection spreads from human to human through direct, indirect, contaminated objects or surfaces or close contact with infected people via oral, or nasal secretions. These include saliva and respiratory secretions, etc. The virus is stable on plastic and stainless steel material [6]. It can be transmitted through routes other than respiratory droplets, such as through the fecal-oral route.

Asymptomatic individuals pose the high-risk transmission, individuals with undocumented infections, people with mild symptoms, and people contagious during the incubation period. The end of the SARS-CoV-2 and COVID-19 pandemic will depend on multiple factors, including social distancing, masks, vaccination, treatment effectiveness, herd immunity, etc. The general physiological measures to prevent the spread of COVID-19 include isolation of infected individuals, quarantine, preventing close contact, and travel restrictions. Nevertheless, the main question still stands: how long will these restrictions last, and when will this pandemic finally come to an end?

Social Distancing and Spread of SARS-CoV-2

Social distancing is also known as "physical distancing," which means keeping a safe space usually defined as about 6 feet (2 meters) between yourself and other people who are not from your household. The social distancing practice, in combination with other preventive measures, reduces the spread of COVID-19. The spread of SARS-CoV-2 infection is mainly found among people in close contact for a long duration. The spread of the virus happens when an infected person coughs, sneezes, or talks, and droplets from their mouth or nose enter into the environment. The virus can easily affect nearby people via direct or indirect contact [7]. The novel coronavirus is an invisible enemy [8]; hence, controlling its spread of disease is no easy task. Symptomatic people can go into quarantine upon recognizing their symptoms. However, asymptomatic people, who are mainly children and young adults who are asymptomatic or have mild symptoms, are unaware that they are infected. Since they do not know to quarantine, minimizing the spread of the disease becomes difficult.

The literature demonstrates that the percentage of asymptomatic cases is about 24.2%. The studies, and results from different prediction models, indicate that undocumented and asymptomatic patients range from 9.2% to 69%. The findings from 565 Japanese people who came from Wuhan, China, showed that five out of eight were positive without clinical features: "asymptomatic" [9].

Asymptomatic patients are contagious and, thus, a potential source of transmission of COVID-19. These asymptomatic patients with COVID-19 tend to be more socially active, quickly moving from one place to another place. The younger asymptomatic patients are usually more active and have more social contacts and are a potential primary source of transmission of

COVID-19 [9]. The use of masks is the best way to minimize the chances of contamination from both asymptomatic and symptomatic patients. Worldwide, policymakers established policies of wearing masks, social distancing, and discouraging gatherings to protect people from this highly contagious disease.

Vaccines and the End of the COVID-19 Pandemic

A year after the appearance of the first case of SARS-CoV-2, the authorizations of the Pfizer vaccine on December 11, 2020 [10] and Moderna vaccine on December 18, 2020 [11] have brought forth a global ray of optimism for concluding the fight against COVID-19. The Food and Drug Authority (FDA) has authorized, on an emergency basis, the Pfizer/BioNTech and Moderna vaccines. These two vaccines can protect by the formation of antibodies to provide immunity against the SARS-CoV-2 infection, with humoral and possibly cellular immunity, which has led to great hope for ending the COVID-19 pandemic.

Table 9.I: Comparison between pharmacology, indications, and adverse effects of Pfizer/BioNTech and Moderna Vaccines.

Characteristics	Pfizer/BioNTech Vaccine	Moderna Vaccine
General name	Pfizer/BioNTech Vaccine [12]	Moderna Vaccine [13]
Generic name	Tozinameran, brand name Comirnaty [12]	Moderna COVID-19 Vaccine [13
Manufacturer	Pfizer, Inc and BioNTech [12]	ModernaTX, Inc [13]
Type of vaccine	mRNA (BNT162b2) [12]	mRNA (mRNA-1273) [13]
FDA Approval	Emergency authorization Dec 11, 2020 [12]	Emergency authorization Dec 18, 2020 [13]
Dose	Each dose contains 30 µg (0.3 mL) [14,15]	Each dose contains 50 µg (0.5 mL) [16,17].
Number of injections	Two shots, given 21 days apart [14]	Two shots, given 28 days apart [16]
Route of administration	Intramuscular-deltoid muscle [12]	Intramuscular-deltoid muscle [13]

Booster shots	Further research is needed to determine whether shots will be required over the year to maintain immunity or be given annually like the flu shot.	Further research is needed to determine whether booster shots will be required over the year to maintain immunity or be given annually like the flu shot.
The age group for vaccination	Sixteen years of age and older [14].	Eighteen years of age and older [17].
Effectiveness	95% in preventing the SARS-COV-2 infection [14]	94.5% in preventing the SARS-COV-2 infection [16]
Approximate cost per dose	Freely available in many developed nations. However, $19.50 per dose excluding taxes, distribution, storage, and health care services cost [18].	Freely available in many developed nations. However, $32-37 per dose excluding taxes, distribution, storage, and health care services cost [18].
Storage	Multiple-dose vials are stored between -80°C to -60°C (-112°F to -76°F). Thaw and store undiluted vials in the refrigerator [2°C to 8°C (35°F to 46°F)] for up to 5 days (120 hours) [19]	Multiple-dose vials are stored between -25° to-15°C (-13° to 5°F). Vials can be stored refrigerated between 2° to 8°C (36° to 46°F) for up to 30 days before first use [20].
Transportation / Distribution	Complicated, complex distribution, particularly in low-income and hot climate countries.	Complicated, complex distribution, particularly in low-income and hot climate countries.
Immunogenicity	Immunogenicity persisted over a median of 2 months [14]	Immunogenicity continued for at least three months. 119 days after the first vaccination and 90 days after the second vaccination [16]

The available evidence supports the conclusion that both vaccines are beneficial but may cause some adverse effects, including pain, redness, or swelling at the site of vaccine shots, nausea, vomiting, fever, fatigue, headache, muscle pain, itching, chills, and joint pain. Rare cases may include anaphylactic reactions as well.

However, differences between the two arise when their cost factors, storage requirements, and beneficial or adverse effects are considered. The Pfizer vaccine is significantly less costly than the Moderna vaccine, and they cost $19.50 and $32-37, respectively [18]. While certain developed nations are vaccinating their citizens free of charge, others are charging the public and must consider whether the vaccine is affordable for all the citizens because the health and lives of all individuals of a society are equally important. Universal vaccination is an excellent way to reach herd immunity. Special consideration must be taken by low-income countries where the average person can afford the vaccine or not. However, despite its lower cost [19], the Pfizer vaccine may face some storage issues, especially in developing countries facing an energy crisis. Simultaneously, the Moderna vaccine is stored at a relatively much higher temperature of between -25° to -15°C [20] that is easier to maintain. This temperature requirement can pose a challenge to low-income countries, many of which also face an energy crisis, as to how they will manage such low storage temperature conditions to ensure the promising results of both the vaccines, especially the Pfizer vaccine, which, although cheaper, requires much lower and more challenging to maintain storage temperatures. The published data has shown that both vaccines elicit a similar humoral response and reports no difference in cellular immunity. There is, however, some preliminary evidence that Pfizer's COVID-19 vaccine may trigger more robust CD8 T-cell responses than Moderna's vaccine [21]. This cellular response might provide added protection against infection.

Compared to the Pfizer vaccine, the Moderna vaccine is easier to transport and store because it is less temperature-sensitive. Clinical trials were conducted under widely varying conditions; hence, adverse effects cannot be directly compared with another vaccine [22]. There are few concerns about these vaccines since the global population will take a minimum period of more than one year to provide vaccination and achieve a target of 65-75% herd immunity.

Herd Immunity and the COVID-19 Pandemic

The world is currently facing a threatening coronavirus pandemic situation, which began 18 years ago, when SARS-CoV-1, a coronavirus, was a major pandemic of the new millennium [2]. Eighteen years ago, in March 2003, many people were infected with a mortality rate of 9%. In a few months, SARS-CoV-1 was detected in several countries. Researchers pointed out that the virus could gain mutations favoring human infection. After 18 years since the SARS-CoV-1 epidemic, the world is facing the most challenging pandemic since the Spanish flu in 1918. The current pandemic has affected over 107 million people and caused over 2.3 million deaths worldwide [4].

The SARS-CoV-2 infection is highly contagious and dangerous, and many queries are related to immunity; how long does the immunological memory last, and how the entire world will cope with this long-lasting pandemic needs to be clarified. Regarding community protection, acquiring herd immunity or community immunity is one modality to minimize and stop the disease spreading [23].

"Herd immunity," also called "community immunity, population immunity, or social immunity," is a form of indirect protection from any infectious disease that occurs when a large percentage of a population has become immune to an infection, whether through previous infectious exposure or vaccination. Herd or community immunity develops once a major part of the population in a specific region becomes immune to a particular disease. Herd immunity also stops the spreading of diseases. The infection rate decreases and the disease is gradually eradicated. When herd immunity is present, immunological memory will be sustained by memory immune clones after recovery from an infection. If another exposure to the same antigen occurs, then it protects the individual from the same infection. The Zika virus outbreak in Brazil was eradicated after about 63% of the population was exposed to the virus, and herd immunity was achieved [24]. Another example is eliminating the poliomyelitis virus and its spread due to vaccination [25]. For understanding the basic concept of herd immunity and the hypothesis about the end of any contagious diseases, it is essential to comprehend reproduction numbers.

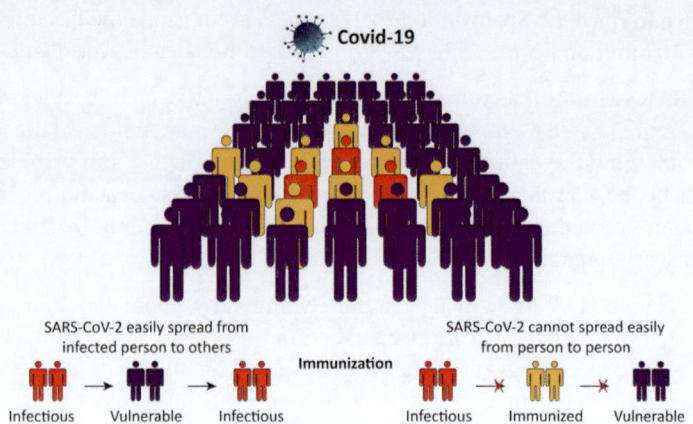

Figure 9.2: Role of herd immunity

The transmission of viruses can be investigated by the basic reproduction number (R0). The R number is known as "naught or zero" (R0) or the adequate reproduction number (Re). R0 is an important parameter to formulate possible preventive measures. The R number measures the average number of new cases generated per typical infectious case. The R number of the virus in the pandemic's epicenter was decreased below the vital threshold value of 1.0 [26, 27]. An R0 above 1 demonstrates that the number of infected people is likely to increase, and an R0 less than 1 shows that transmission is expected to decrease and end. This number demonstrates that if a person who is infected in turn infects less than one person, then the outbreak will be reduced. An R-value of 0.5 shows that 10 infected people can infect five, who would then infect another 2.5. In contrast, a Re above 1 would mean that the outbreak would increase exponentially [27].

The percentage of the population required for a community to reach herd immunity depends on the basic reproduction number (R0). The higher the R_0, the more people are needed to be resistant, in order to achieve herd immunity [28]. There are multiple examples of earlier infectious disease epidemics. In 1918, the Spanish flu pandemic, which spread to one-third of the world's population and had a death toll of up to 50 million, had an R_0 of 1.8 [29]. For SARS-CoV-2, in Wuhan, China, R_0 was calculated, and the mean R_0 for COVID-19 was around 3.28, with a median of 2.79 (2-3). The period for this study was from January 1, 2020, to February 7, 2020 [Liu et al., 2020] [30].

To understand the epidemiological trends of any contagious disease, it is essential to know that herd immunity must be in the range of 50–67% of the population [Liu et al., 2020] [30]. Vaccination is the best way to stop infectious diseases [30]. If the community contains around 64% immunized individuals, the disease will not spread to susceptible ones, and finally, the spreading of the virus will slow down.

In a large metanalysis conducted by Billah et al., 2020 [31], it was estimated that the reproductive number indicates an exponential increase of coronavirus infection. The analysis was based on 29 articles. The estimated summary reproductive number was 2.87 (95% CI, 2.39–3.44). It indicates that worldwide, the COVID-19 pandemic is still spreading. The study was submitted for publication in May 2020 and was published on November 11, 2020, with data collected before the start of vaccination [31]. In another study, Dharmaratne et al., 2020 [32] calculated the R0 of the coronavirus disease COVID-19 in Sri Lanka and described the variation of R, with its implications for the prevention and control of the disease. The authors estimated that the R0 for COVID-19 in Sri Lanka was between 0.93 and 1.23, and the transmissibility R has reduced, indicating that measures implemented have achieved reasonable control of the disease. The vaccination rates, and herd immunity allied data are not known globally. Hence, global epidemiologists have concerns about whether they can appropriately calculate and understand the timeline for a transition toward normalcy.

The Transition Toward Normalcy

Considering the scientific facts, it is difficult to predict the transitioning phase toward normalcy before the detailed global information on vaccination and herd immunity, which must be achieved by more than 65-75 % of the population. COVID-19 will not disappear during this transition but will become a more routine part of the baseline disease burden in society, rather than a current pandemic threat. During this transition, controlling the spread of SARS-CoV2 will require public health measures, including social distancing, use of masks, avoiding public gatherings, COVID-19 testing, and vaccination.

The transition toward normalcy is likely to occur during early 2022 if vaccine doses reach a significant percentage of high-risk elderly individuals by mid-2021. The arrival of spring 2021 in the northern hemisphere should improve the situation [33].

The slow distribution of the vaccines and the spread of additional infectious variants increases the risk of delaying a transition to normalcy. Estimates based on the broadest possible available scientific literature demonstrate that herd immunity might not be reached until the end of 2021. It is a fact that a potentially shorter duration of immunity could prolong the path to the "end." The duration of immunity is very important, and herd immunity to COVID-19 is unlikely to be achieved unless adult vaccination rates approach 65-75 percent. Recent developments suggest that herd immunity will most likely come in late 2021. We can practically hope for an end to this pandemic by the mid-2022.

Conclusion

The war against COVID-19 is far from over in 2021. Current preventive measures and vaccinations are essential to minimize the incidence and mortality of this disease but will not completely eradicate the virus. The community must be educated to adapt and embrace self-discipline to prevent the spreading of SARS-COV-2 infection. Measures such as social distancing, use of masks, and personal hygiene will remain in place until a maximum number of people receive vaccinations worldwide. The science community has succeeded in developing vaccines that have been authorized around the world against SARS-CoV-2. People are receiving vaccinations, and populations are developing herd immunity, but the pandemic has not settled down. Considering current public health policies, self-preventive measures, the use of vaccines, and herd immunity, there is great hope for ending the COVID-19 pandemic by the end of 2022.

References

1. Meo SA, Al-Khlaiwi T, Usmani AM, Meo AS, Klonoff DC, Hoang TD. Biological and epidemiological trends in the prevalence and mortality due to outbreaks of novel coronavirus COVID-19. .J King Saud Univ Sci. 2020 Jun;32(4):2495-2499. doi: 10.1016/j.jksus.2020.04.004.

2. Meo SA, Alhowikan AM, Al-Khlaiwi T, Meo IM, Halepoto DM, Iqbal M, Usmani AM, Hajjar W, Ahmed N. Novel coronavirus 2019-nCoV: prevalence, biological and clinical characteristics comparison with SARS-CoV and MERS-CoV. Eur Rev Med Pharmacol Sci. 2020 Feb;24(4):2012-2019. doi: 10.26355/eurrev_202002_20379.

3.   Anderson RM, Vegvari C, Truscott J, Collyer BS. Challenges in creating herd immunity to SARS-CoV-2 infection by mass vaccination. Lancet. 2020 Nov 21;396(10263):1614-1616. doi: 10.1016/S0140-6736(20)32318-7. Epub 2020 November 4. PMID: 33159850; PMCID: PMC7836302.

4.   World Health Organization, Coronavirus Disease (COVID-19) Dashboard: Available at https://covid19.who.int/ Cited date February 13, 2021.

5.   Prather KA, Wang CC, Schooley RT. Reducing the transmission of SARS-CoV-2. Science. 2020 June 26;368(6498):1422-1424. doi: 10.1126/science.abc6197.

6.   Van Doremalen N, Bushmaker T, Morris DH, Holbrook MG, Gamble A, Williamson BN, Tamin A, Harcourt JL, Thornburg NJ, Gerber SI, Lloyd-Smith JO, de Wit E, Munster VJ. Aerosol and Surface Stability of SARS-CoV-2 as Compared with SARS-CoV-1. N Engl J Med. 2020 April 16;382(16):1564-1567. doi: 10.1056/NEJMc2004973.

7.   Centers for Disease Prevention and Control (CDC). Social distancing. Available at: https://www.cdc.gov/coronavirus/2019-ncov/prevent-getting-sick/social-distancing.html. Cited date February 2, 2021.

8.   Shafi KM, Meo AS, Khalid R. Covid-19: Invisible, Elusive and the Advancing Enemy. Pak J Med Sci. 2020;36(COVID19-S4): S138-S139. doi:10.12669/pjms.36.COVID19-S4.2758

9.   Kronbichler A, Kresse D, Yoon S, Lee KH, Effenberger M, Shin JI. Asymptomatic patients as a source of COVID-19 infections: A systematic review and meta-analysis. Int J Infect Dis. 2020 98:180-186. doi: 10.1016/j.ijid.2020.06.052.

10. US Food and Drug Administration. Pfizer-BioNTech COVID-19 Vaccine. Available at: https://www.fda.gov/emergency-preparedness-and-response/coronavirus-disease-2019-covid-19/pfizer-biontech-covid-19-vaccine. Cited date December 24, 2020.

11. US Food and Drug Ad. Available at: https://www.fda.gov/media/144412/download. Cited date December 24, 2020.

12. Centre for Disease Control Prevention (CDC). Information about the Pfizer-BioNTech COVID-19 Vaccine. Available at: https://www.fda.gov/emergency-preparedness-and-response/coronavirus-disease-2019-covid-19/pfizer-biontech-covid-19-vaccine#additional. Cited dated, December 24, 2020.

13. Centre for Disease Control Prevention (CDC). Information about the Moderna COVID-19 Vaccine. Available https://www.fda.gov/media/144638/download. Cited Date December 24, 2020.

14. Polack FP, Thomas SJ, Kitchin N, Absalon J, Gurtman A, Lockhart S, Perez JL, Pérez Marc G, Moreira ED, Zerbini C, Bailey R, Swanson KA, Roychoudhury S, Koury K, Li P, Kalina WV, Cooper D, Frenck RW Jr, Hammitt LL, Türeci Ö, Nell H, Schaefer A, Ünal S, Tresnan DB, Mather S, Dormitzer PR, Şahin U, Jansen KU, Gruber WC; C4591001 Clinical Trial Group. Safety and Efficacy of the BNT162b2 mRNA Covid-19 Vaccine. N Engl J Med 2020; 383: 2603-2615.

15. Oliver SE, Gargano JW, Marin M, Wallace M, Curran KG, Chamberland M, McClung N, Campos-Outcalt D, Morgan RL, Mbaeyi S, Romero JR, Talbot HK, Lee GM, Bell BP, Dooling K. The Advisory Committee on Immunization Practices' Interim Recommendation for the use of Pfizer-BioNTech COVID-19 Vaccine - United States, December 2020. MMWR Morb Mortal Wkly Rep 2020; 69: 1922-1924.

16. Widge AT, Rouphael NG, Jackson LA, Anderson EJ, Roberts PC, Makhene M, Chappell JD, Denison MR, Stevens LJ, Pruijssers AJ. mRNA-1273 Study Group. The durability of Responses after SARS-CoV-2 mRNA-1273 vaccination. N Engl J Med 2021; 384: 80-82. doi: 10.1056/NEJMc2032195

17. Jackson LA, Anderson EJ, Rouphael NG, Roberts PC, Makhene M, Coler RN, McCullough MP, Chappell JD, Denison MR. mRNA-1273 Study Group. An mRNA Vaccine against SARS-CoV-2 - Preliminary Report. N Engl J Med 2020; 383: 1920-1931.

18. Katie Jennings. Forbes. How much will it cost to get a COVID-19 vaccine? Available at: www.healthline.com/health-news/how-much-will-it-cost-to-get-a-covid-19-vaccine#What-we-know-about-distribution-and-administration-costs. Cited date December 24, 2020

19. Pfizer-BioNTech COVID-19 Vaccine. Fact Sheet. Available at: https://www.fda.gov/media/144413/download. Cited date December 25, 2020.

20. Moderna COVID-19 Vaccine. Fact Sheet. Available at: Mohttps://www.idsociety.org/covid-19-real-time-learning-network/vaccines/moderna-covid-19-vaccine/. Cited date December 25, 2020.

21. Nick Paul Taylor. Pfizer reports strong T-cell response to the COVID-19 vaccine. Fierce Biotech. Available at: https://www.fiercebiotech.com/biotech/pfizer-reports-strong-t-cell-response-to-covid-19-vaccine. Cited date December 26, 2020.

22. Meo SA, Bukhari IA, Akram J, Meo AS, Klonoff DC.COVID-19 vaccines: comparison of biological, pharmacological characteristics and adverse effects of Pfizer/BioNTech and Moderna Vaccines. Eur Rev Med Pharmacol Sci. 2021 Feb;25(3):1663-1669.

23. Monica Neagu. The bumpy road to achieve herd immunity in COVID-19. Journal of Immunoassay and Immunochemistry. 2020; 928-945. doi.org/10.1080/15321819.2020.1833919

24. Carvalho MS, Freitas LP, Cruz OG, Brasil P, Bastos LS. Association of past Dengue Fever Epidemics with the Risk of Zika Microcephaly at the Population Level in Brazil. Sci. Rep. 2020, 10, 1752. DOI: 10.1038/s41598-020-58407-7.

25. Bandyopadhyay AS, Macklin GR. Final Frontiers of the Polio Eradication Endgame. Curr. Opin. Infect. Dis. 2020, 33(5), 404-410. DOI: 10.1097/QCO.0000000000000667.

26. Rahman B, Sadraddin E, Porreca A. The basic reproduction number of SARS-CoV-2 in Wuhan is about to die out; how about the rest of the world? Rev Med Virol. 2020 Jul;30(4):e2111. doi: 10.1002/rmv.2111.

27. Mahase E. Covid-19: What is the R number? BMJ 2020; 369. doi.org/10.1136/bmj.m1891.

28. Kirtimaan S. COVID-19: Herd Immunity and Convalescent Plasma Transfer Therapy. J. Med. Virol. 2020. DOI: 10.1002/jmv.25870.

29. Biggerstaff, M.; Cauchemez, S.; Reed, C.; Gambhir, M.; Finelli, L. Estimates of the Reproduction Number for Seasonal, Pandemic, and Zoonotic Influenza: A Systematic Review of the Literature. BMC Infect. Dis. 2014, 14, 480. DOI: 10.1186/1471-2334-14-480.

30. Liu, Y.; Gayle, A. A.; Wilder-Smith, A.; Rocklov, J. The Reproductive Number of COVID-19 Is Higher Compared to SARS Coronavirus. J. Travel Med. 2020, 27(2), taaa021. DOI: 10.1093/jtm/taaa021.

31. Billah M.A, Miah M.M, Khan M.N (2020). A Reproductive number of coronavirus: A systematic review and meta-analysis based on global level evidence. PLoS ONE 15(11): e0242128. https://doi. org/10.1371/journal.pone.0242128.

32. Dharmaratne S, Sudaraka S, Abeyagunawardena I, Manchanayake K, Kothalawala M, Gunathunga W. Estimation of the basic reproduction number (R0) novel coronavirus disease in Sri Lanka. Virol J. 2020; 17: 144. doi: 10.1186/s12985-020-01411-0.

33. Charumilind S, Craven M, Lamb J, Sabow A, Wilson M. When will the COVID-19 pandemic end. Available at: https://www.mckinsey.com/industries/healthcare-systems-and-services/our-insights/when-will-the-covid-19-pandemic-end. Cited date February 4, 2021.